Color Atlas of High Resolution Manometry

Color Atlas of High Resolution Manometry

Edited by

Jeffrey Conklin, MD
GI Motility Program

Mark Pimentel, MD, FRCP(C)
Cedars-Sinai Medical Center

Edy Soffer, MD
Los Angeles, California, USA

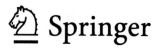 Springer

Editors
Jeffrey Conklin, MD
GI Motility Program

Mark Pimentel, MD, FRCP(C)
Cedars-Sinai Medical Center

Edy Soffer, MD
Los Angeles, California, USA

ISBN: 978-0-387-88292-5   e-ISBN: 978-0-387-88295-6
DOI: 10.1007/978-0-387-88295-6

Library of Congress Control Number: 2008935896

This book is dedicated to the memory of Ray E Clouse MD, an outstanding educator and clinician. His research and foresight laid the foundations for the development of high-resolution manometry.

Acknowledgement

We would like to thank Laura Hwang for her assistance in assembling the components of this book.

About the Authors

Jeffrey Conklin, MD
Director, Esophageal Program
Cedars-Sinai Medical Center
Los Angeles, California

Mark Pimentel, MD, FRCP(C)
Director, GI Motility Program
Cedars-Sinai Medical Center
Los Angeles, California

Edy Soffer, MD
Co-Director, GI Motility Program
Cedars-Sinai Medical Center
Los Angeles, California

Contents

Acknowledgement vii

About the Authors ix

1 Introduction to High-Resolution Manometry 1
   1.1. High-Resolution Manometry: How Does It Work? 2

2 Esophageal Manometry 11
   2.1. Normal High-Resolution Esophageal Manometry 12
         2.1.1. Respiratory Variations in the Body
                 of the Esophagus 12
         2.1.2. Transition Zone 13
         2.1.3. Pressure Inversion Point 15
         2.1.4. Lower Esophageal Sphincter 15
         2.1.5. Normal Bolus Pressure 16
         2.1.6. Peristalsis 17
         2.1.7. Gastric Pressures 17
   2.2. Abnormal High-Resolution Esophageal Manometry 17
         2.2.1. Achalasia 17
         2.2.2. Diffuse Esophageal Spasm 25
         2.2.3. Nutcracker Esophagus 32
         2.2.4. Hiatal Hernia 32
         2.2.5. Gastroesophageal Reflux Disease
                 and Lower Esophageal Sphincter 32
         2.2.6. Scleroderma 32
         2.2.7. Ineffective Esophageal Motility 32
         2.2.8. Cricopharyngeal Bar 40
         2.2.9. Other Esophageal Observations with
                 High-Resolution Manometry 40
   2.3. Troubleshooting in High-Resolution Manometry
         of the Esophagus 51
         2.3.1. Folded Catheter 51
         2.3.2. Failed Sensor Bank 51
         2.3.3. Air in the Sheath 55

3   Gastric/Small Bowel Manometry 59
   3.1. Normal Gastric and Small Bowel
      High-Resolution Manometry 59
      3.1.1 Fasting State 60
      3.1.2. Fed State 62

4   Anorectal Manometry 71
   4.1. Normal High-Resolution Anorectal Manometry 71
      4.1.1. Normal Anal Sphincter 71
      4.1.2. Cough Reflex 80
      4.1.3. Oscillating Pressure Waves 80
      4.1.4. Anoanal Reflex 80
      4.1.5. Rectal Response to Balloon Distention 80
   4.2. Abnormal High-Resolution Anorectal Manometry 80
      4.2.1. Dyssynergic Defecation 80
      4.2.2. Hirschsprung's Disease 80
      4.2.3. Troubleshooting 88

Index 89

1

Introduction to High-Resolution Manometry

Various techniques, such as the measurement of pressure events within the gut, facilitate assessment of gastrointestinal motor functions. Systems for the recording of intraluminal pressure events have evolved from simple balloons to perfused and solid-state catheters. Display and analysis methods have evolved from strip chart recorders to computerized systems. Each advance has brought a better understanding of gastrointestinal motor physiology. Perfused manometric systems have been the norm for the past two to three decades. A new manometric technique, high-resolution manometry (HRM), promises a better description of complex gastrointestinal motions.

This introduction reviews the underlying concepts and technical development of HRM, discusses how it differs from conventional manometric techniques, and compares and contrasts the information provided by HRM with that obtained by standard techniques. Such comparisons highlight how HRM helps, and where traditional manometry fails in providing detailed information on gut motor function.

Over the last few decades, most medical centers and office-based practices conducting motility testing have used water-perfused systems. These systems consist of a multilumen catheter (Fig. 1.1) connected to an array of pressure transducers, a pneumohydraulic pump to provide the continuous flow of water, and a display system. The pneumohydraulic pump drives water through the very narrow channels of the catheter at a constant low rate, but under high pressure. Each channel of the catheter is connected to a separate pressure transducer. Any interference with the flow of water from any of the various channels by lumen occluding contractions raises the pressure in the corresponding channel. Pressure transducers continuously monitor pressures in the channels. Pressure information is transmitted to a computer, where it is digitized, analyzed, and displayed on a video monitor. The manometric output of such a catheter array and recording system is shown in Fig. 1.2.

While they are robust and accurate, most perfused systems can accommodate rather few recording channels because of constraints on catheter size. This limits the amount of information obtained, particularly from sphincteric regions. High-resolution manometry does not suffer from such limitations.

J. Conklin, *Color Atlas of High Resolution Manometry*,
DOI: 10.1007/978-0-387-88295-6_1, © Springer Science+Business Media, LLC 2009

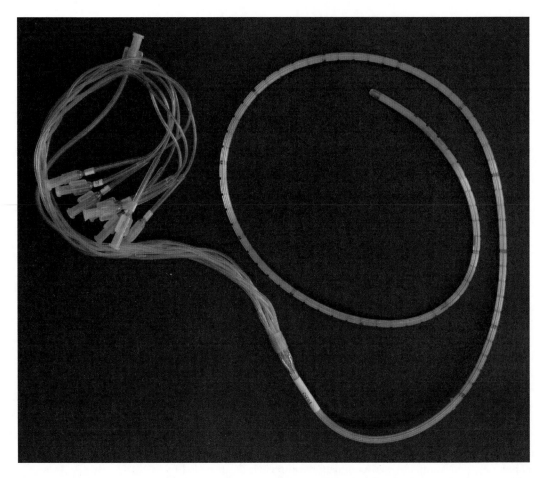

Fig. 1.1. Water-perfused manometry catheters like the one pictured are a bundle of thin polyvinyl tubes, with an outward facing opening (side hole) in each tube. The side holes function as point pressure sensors. They are typically configured at 3- to 5-cm intervals along the catheter. A low-compliance, pneumohydraulic pump slowly perfuses each of the tubes, and the pressure in each is converted to an electrical signal by a volume-displacement transducer. Pressure recorded by the system increases when water flowing through the side hole is impeded by radial contraction of the gut wall at the side hole. Information about gastrointestinal motor function may be lost with this technique because the side holes are widely spaced and sense in only one direction around the catheter circumference.

1.1. High-Resolution Manometry: How Does It Work?

Developments in both software and hardware made high-resolution recording possible. Miniaturization of strain gauges facilitated the incorporation of multiple, closely spaced pressure sensors in the catheter (Fig. 1.3). This HRM catheter contains 36 sensors, each one averaging pressures from 12 positions in its circumference. The sensors are spaced 1 cm apart, spanning a length of 35 cm. In the esophagus, this enables simultaneous recording from all segments, including the sphincteric regions, pharynx, and stomach, without the need to reposition the catheter during the study, the so-called pull-through technique.

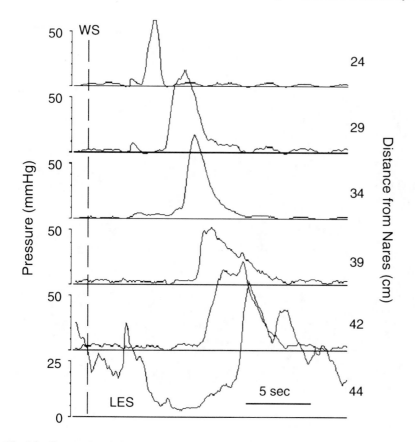

Fig. 1.2. Conventional manometric recording. This is an example of normal esophageal motor function as recorded with a conventional water-perfused manometry system. Time is on the x-axis. The numbers to the right indicate the distance of the side-hole sensors from the nares, and the numbers to the left indicate the pressure scale at each side-hole location. Occurrence of a wet swallow is indicated by WS. The most distal sensor (bottom trace) is in the lower esophageal sphincter (LES), a zone of high pressure near the gastroesophageal (GE) junction that transiently diminishes with swallowing. The five pressure sensing sites above the LES record a peristaltic pressure wave. Manometry systems of this type cannot, in general, simultaneously record from all constituent components of the esophagus, that is, the LES, esophageal body, and upper esophageal sphincter (UES).

The second major development involves the software used to analyze pressure data, and the application of color contours to depict intraluminal pressure. Figure 1.4 provides an explanation of how the HRM image is derived from pressure data. A comparison of conventional manometric data (Fig. 1.2) with those obtained by HRM (Fig. 1.4F) makes it clear that the rich detail of color contour plots provides a great deal more information and better assessment of motor events in the entire gut segment being studied. Use of the color contour also enables the reader to change the gain (pressure–color relationship) to appreciate subtle findings (Fig. 1.5). Isobaric contour lines can highlight areas of similar pressure (Fig. 1.6).

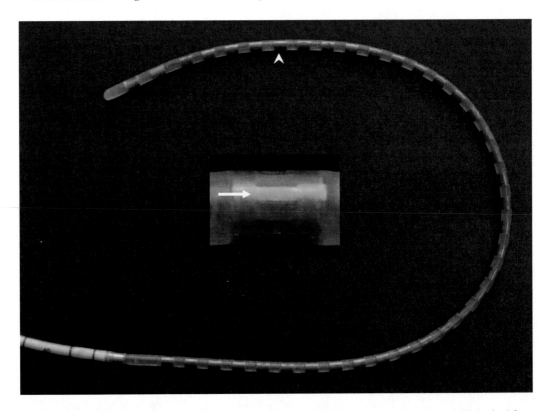

Fig. 1.3. High-resolution manometry catheter. The high-resolution manometry catheter pictured here is 4.2 mm in diameter and consists of 36 circumferential, solid-state, pressure sensors (copper colored bands, *arrowhead*). Sensors are spaced at 1-cm intervals, from center to center. This gives the catheter a recording segment of 35 cm. Each individual sensor (magnified at center) detects pressure from 12 loci (*arrow*) around its circumference. Computer processing of the signals coming from pressure sensing elements allows average circumferential pressures over the entire 35-cm recording segment to be displayed in real time and recorded for subsequent analysis.

Fig. 1.4. Transformation of manometric pressure into a topographic (color contour) plot of high-resolution manometry. Conventional manometry systems record and display intraluminal pressures from sensors that are relatively widely spaced, usually at 3- to 5-cm intervals. (A) This recording was made with a high-resolution manometry catheter and recording system (Manoscan™, Sierra Scientific Instruments), but it is displayed in the line mode so it looks like a conventional esophageal manometry recording. Nine of 36 recording channels were chosen for display to mimic what is seen with conventional manometry systems. Channels were selected to record simultaneously from the pharynx to the stomach. Pressure is on the y-axis, time is on the x-axis, and pressure tracings are stacked vertically with the proximal sensor at the top and the distal sensor at the bottom. This gives a two-dimensional display. The numbers to the right of the graphic indicate sensor spacing relative to the nares. The tracing labeled UES is from the upper esophageal sphincter, and that labeled LES is from the lower esophageal sphincter. WS indicates the timing of a wet swallow. The esophageal peristaltic pressure wave, and relaxation of the UES and LES are seen in this recording. These tracings can be displayed three-dimensionally by stacking them horizontally rather than vertically (B). Pressure remains on the y-axis and time on the x-axis. Sensor position is now on the z-axis with the most distal sensor (gastric) at the front and the most proximal sensor (pharynx) at the back. New high-resolution manometry (HRM) systems record intraluminal pressures circumferentially at 1-cm intervals over a 35-cm recording segment. (C) A display of data from all 36-pressure sensors on the HRM catheter during the same wet swallow depicted in panels A and B. The added pressure information provides better spatial resolution of esophageal motor function. (D) Time and pressure contour lines are applied to the tracings with isobaric pressure lines at 5-mmHg intervals. (E) Colors are assigned to pressures to form a color contour plot. Cooler colors represent lower pressures and warmer colors represent higher pressures. Rotating this plot so that you look down

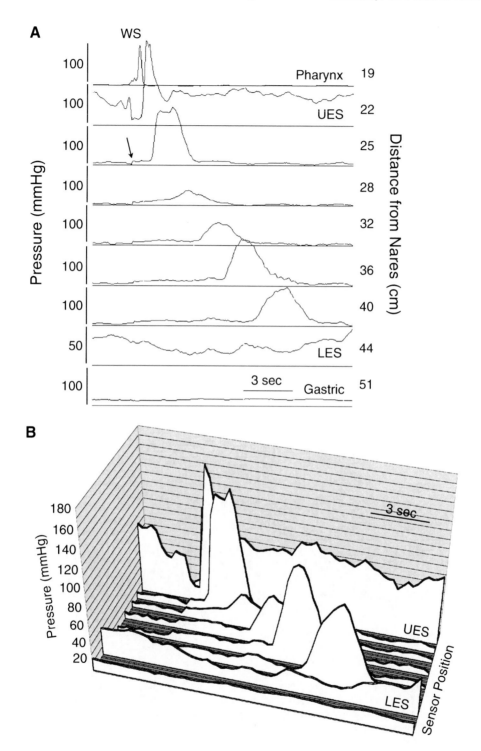

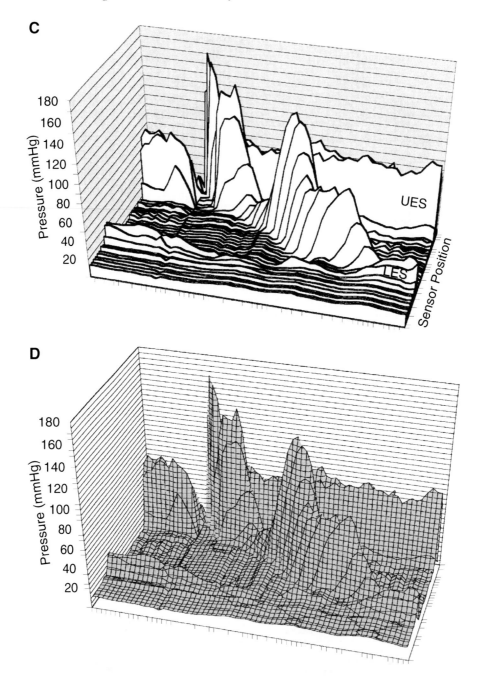

Fig. 1.4. (continued) on it from directly above produces the color display seen in the contour mode of the HRM recording (F). This display technique collapses the pressure axis of the three-dimensional color contour to a two-dimensional surface in which pressure is represented by color, sensor location is on the y-axis, and time is on the x-axis. Resting UES and LES pressures are seen in the color contour plot as horizontal bands of color that are several centimeters wide. Their hues indicate pressures that are greater than in the adjacent pharynx, esophagus, or stomach. Opening of the UES and LES relaxation are depicted as changes of color to hues that represent a lower pressure: UES pressure approximates that in the esophagus (*), and LES pressure approximates that in the stomach (**). Notice that the LES relaxes shortly after opening of the UES. The peristaltic pressure wave is portrayed as a diagonal band of color running from the UES to the LES. It is of relatively high pressure in the striated muscle segment, diminishes over the transition zone, and increases in amplitude in the smooth muscle esophagus. Pressure in the swallowed bolus (intrabolus pressure) is represented by a small simultaneous rise in intraesophageal pressure (*arrow*). It occurs shortly after initiation of the wet swallow, and

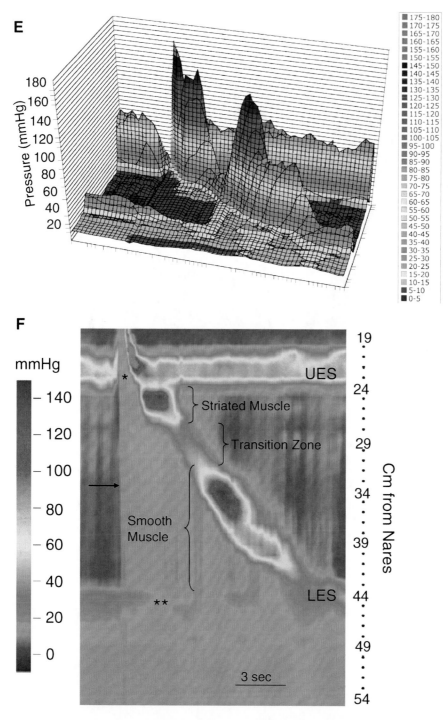

Fig. 1.4. (continued) remains elevated ahead of the peristaltic pressure wave. The intrabolus pressure can also be seen in panel A (*arrow*), but the pressure change is subtle. Intraesophageal pressure drops after the peristaltic pressure wave passes (return to a darker blue color), indicating bolus clearance from the esophagus. Current high-resolution manometry hardware and software allow switching back and forth between the line mode, which looks like a conventional manometric line tracing, and the contour mode, which displays data as a color encoded isocontour plot. Comparisons between these modes will be made throughout this book.

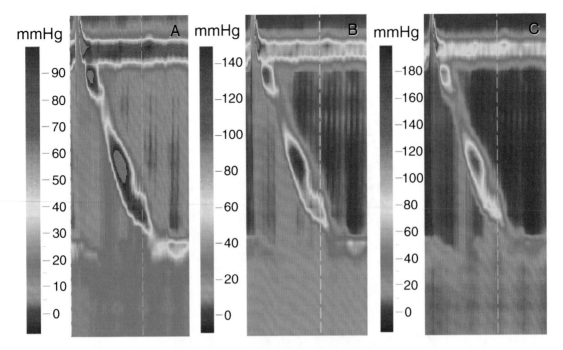

Fig. 1.5. Changing the amplification of high-resolution color contour. As with standard manometry systems, the amplification or gain of the HRM system can be changed. High-amplitude pressure events can be brought into range by decreasing the amplification, and low-amplitude pressure phenomena can be made more visible by increasing it. Altering the amplification changes the height of pressure waves on a standard line tracing, and the colors of the HRM color contour. In this figure, the same pressure data are displayed at a full-scale range of 100 mmHg (A), 150 mmHg (B), and 200 mmHg (C). The color bar correlating color with pressure for each contour is seen to the left of each panel. The appearance of the color contour depends very much on the scale chosen. The bright pink color in A indicates that the pressure is out of range (>100 mmHg), and is brought into range by changing to a full scale of 150 mmHg. To avoid confusion, it is prudent to begin each analysis at a standard range; we choose 150 mmHg. This allows observers to calibrate their eye to a set color/pressure relationship. The gain can then be changed to highlight subtle variations in pressure or bring high pressures into range.

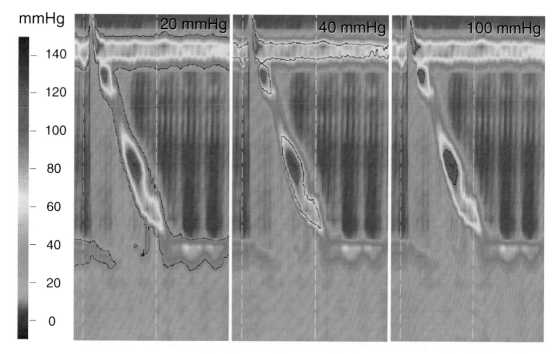

Fig. 1.6. Isobaric pressure contour lines. Isobaric contour lines (black lines) are used to determine at which locations in the color contour plot the pressure is the same. They are akin to contour lines depicting altitude in topographical maps. The pressure, like altitude, is higher inside the contour line and lower outside. In this figure, the same pressure data are displayed at a full-scale range of 150 mmHg (color bar), with isobaric pressure lines drawn at 20, 60, and 100 mmHg.

While this brief introduction to the technique of HRM has focused on the esophagus, the benefits apply equally to recordings from other segments of the gut. High-resolution manometry, while providing numeric data on pressure events in all parts of the gut, begins to provide the opportunity for pattern recognition. The following chapters show some patterns seen with HRM that correspond to normal motility and to disease states.

Esophageal Manometry

Difficulty of access has always limited study of the gut in all its functions. The relative ease of access to the esophagus makes esophageal motor function the area best studied. Also, some of the most common gastrointestinal complaints, such as gastroesophageal reflux disease (GERD), originate from this part of the gut.

It seems intuitive that since the esophagus is so readily accessible and well studied, there would be little new to learn from the investigation of the esophagus. Actually, however, high-resolution manometry (HRM) has already added much to our understanding of esophageal disorders.

A primary benefit of HRM in the esophagus is the ease with which it can be performed. Previous techniques for manometry of the esophagus required multiple maneuvers to position the pressure channels of the catheter in the lower esophageal sphincter (LES). An example of such a maneuver is the so-called station pull-through technique. Since the pressure-sensing channels of water-perfused catheter systems are spaced widely apart, the catheter must be pulled gradually across the LES to appreciate its entire length and the maximal pressure it generates. Furthermore, relaxation of the LES is difficult to observe convincingly because water-perfused catheters are stationary in the LES and, during swallows, esophageal shortening might result in proximal displacement of the LES, giving a false impression of relaxation. Assessment of the upper esophageal sphincter (UES) is also unsatisfactory for many of the same reasons. Sleeve catheters resolved only some of these difficulties.

With HRM of the esophagus, none of these problems exist. The catheter and its 36 channels straddle the entire esophagus simultaneously, so there is no need to move the catheter. Esophageal shortening can be seen without moving the catheter, and the closely spaced sensors provide accurate information on the function of the sphincters. Table 2.1 summarizes some of the important differences between conventional and high-resolution manometry, pertaining to the esophagus.

In this chapter, features of normal and abnormal esophageal manometry are described using the technique of HRM. As will be evident, the color images of manometry using this system provide both quantitative and qualitative information and provide for pattern recognition.

J. Conklin, *Color Atlas of High Resolution Manometry*,
DOI: 10.1007/978-0-387-88295-6_2, © Springer Science+Business Media, LLC 2009

Table 2.1. Benefits of high-resolution manometry compared to conventional manometry for the esophagus.

Conventional manometry	High-resolution manometry
Need to move catheter for LES in most systems	Catheter stays in one position
Water-perfused systems are multicomponent and cumbersome	Solid state and direct interface with stand alone system
Low fidelity	High fidelity
Waveforms only	Color contour
LES measurements complex; some use sleeves, others need station pull-through technique	No need for pull-through technique, and if desired can create an electronic sleeve for LES determination
Hard to find hiatal hernias	Hiatal hernias are immediately visible
Water-perfused catheters are stiff and more uncomfortable	Soft and comfortable
Multiple maneuvers mean a longer test duration	Procedure is quicker since no position changes are needed
Large gaps between pressure channels (most are 5 cm apart); may miss findings	Array of 36 channels straddle the entire esophagus; sees the entire organ

LES, lower esophageal sphincter.

2.1. Normal High-Resolution Esophageal Manometry

As already mentioned, examination of sphincteric activity is easier with HRM. Pressure sensors extend from the hypopharynx to the stomach, straddling both the UES and the LES. Fig. 1.4F (see Chapter 1) depicts a single swallow. The UES is easily visualized as a band of pressure near the top of the figure, and its length can be measured. It is easy to observe the opening of the UES by the change in color to one similar to esophageal resting pressure. Contraction of the striated muscle is observed below the UES, followed by a transition zone between the striated muscle region and the smooth muscle region, which is characterized by low amplitude or no peristalsis. The amplitude of peristaltic activity increases in the smooth muscle esophagus. The LES is seen near the bottom of the image. Its relaxation is observed shortly after swallowing as a drop in pressure to approximate intragastric pressure. A computer algorithm that functions somewhat like a Dent sleeve estimates residual LES pressure. How this electronic or eSleeveTM (Sierra Scientific Instruments) functions is described in figure 2.1. So much detail is provded in the color contour, that pharyngeal measurements are vivid to the point where bolus transfer mechanisms can be seen, as in Fig. 2.1. In fact, a rapid, propulsive pharyngeal pressure wave is seen ahead of the relaxation, propelling the water bolus into the esophagus. This is considered an oropharyngeal bolus transfer event.

2.1.1. Respiratory Variations in the Body of the Esophagus

In Fig. 2.2A, respiratory variations in pressure appear in a record displayed as a conventional manometry. These are clearly visible as subtle color changes on HRM (Fig. 2.2B). These color changes are due to variations in intrathoracic pressure. The typical blue color of resting intraesophageal pressure darkens with inspiration, indicating a lower pressure, and lightens with exhalation, indicating a rise in pressure. This finding assists in localizing the diaphragm,

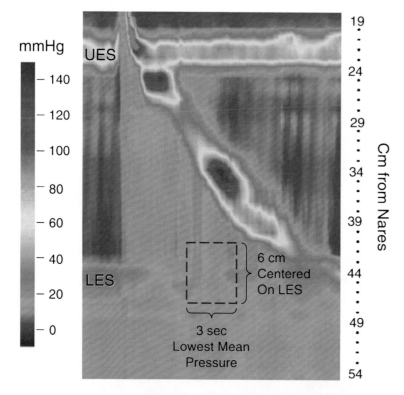

Fig. 2.1. Measurement of residual lower esophageal sphincter (LES) pressure. Residual LES pressure is the lowest LES pressure recorded relative to intragastric pressure during swallow-induced LES relaxation. It is used to determine whether the LES relaxes completely. The most reliable way to measure residual LES pressure with perfused manometry catheters is use the Dent sleeve. When properly positioned across the LES, the sleeve sensor measures pressure simultaneously over a 6-cm segment and ensures continuous measurement of LES pressure as the esophagus shortens during swallowing. It avoids artifacts produced by a point sensor dropping into the stomach, which can be interpreted LES relaxation. A software algorithm using pressure data from the high-resolution manometry catheter was devised to mimic the Dent sleeve. This electronic sleeve (eSleeveTM, Sierra Scientific Instruments) is a virtual Dent sleeve.

since intraabdominal pressure fluctuates inversely to intrathoracic pressure with respiration.

2.1.2. Transition Zone

In normal people, manometry often shows a short zone of low pressure, called the transition zone, between the upper third and distal two thirds of the esophageal body (Fig. 1.4F). In conventional manometry, it is often difficult to identify this phenomenon. The transition zone is the region over which the esophageal musculature changes from striated to smooth muscle.

The reason for this gap in pressure is not clear. In normal subjects the length of the transition zone varies widely and is only evident on high-resolution manometry. Although a gap is expected, the size and position of the normal gap, based on high-resolution manometry, remain to be determined.

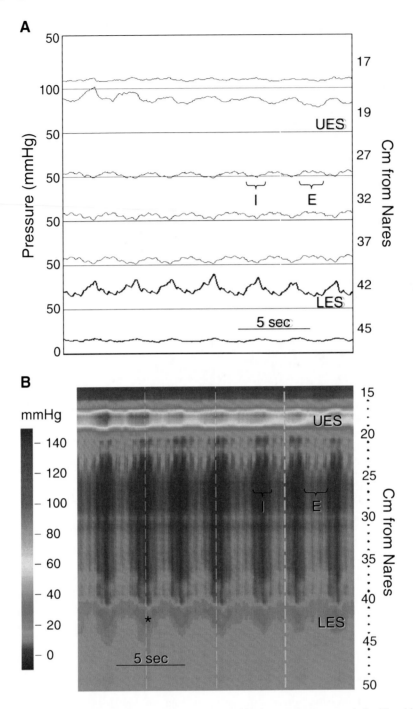

Fig. 2.2. High-resolution manometry of the esophagus at rest. (A) A manometry recorded with a high-resolution manometry (HRM) system, but displayed in line mode as a conventional manometry. It demonstrates a typical recording of the esophagus at rest. The sensor at 17 cm from the nares is in the pharynx, the sensor at 19 cm is in the upper esophageal sphincter (UES), and the sensor at 24 cm is in the LES. Those at 27, 32, and 37 cm are in the esophagus, and the one at 45 cm is intragastric. Inspiration is indicated by I and expiration by E. Pressure becomes more negative in the esophagus during inspiration and more positive during expiration, indicating that the sensors are intrathoracic. It becomes more positive with inspiration and more negative with expiration at the LES (42 cm) and intragastric recording sites, indicating the LES and stomach are below the diaphragm. (B) The same pressure data are displayed as a high-resolution color contour. The catheter was positioned to simultaneously

2.1.3. Pressure Inversion Point

The pressure inversion point (PIP) (also called the respiratory inversion point) is produced by diaphragmatic movement during respiration. Because deep inspiration easily reveals the PIP on conventional manometry, it is often used as a landmark to locate the approximate location of the LES. However, in the case of a small hiatal hernia, this landmark may deceive all but the most experienced gastroenterologists who perform esophageal manometry. Fig. 2.2A demonstrates what the PIP looks like in a record from conventional traditional manometry. There is very little difficulty in the detection of the PIP using high-resolution manometry. However, in Fig. 2.2B, one must learn to recognize the color contour appearance of this phenomenon.

Thus far, little or no work has been done using high-resolution manometry as a means of detecting intrathoracic pressure in pulmonary disease. One might expect deep negative excursions in restrictive lung disease, for example.

2.1.4. Lower Esophageal Sphincter

The LES, a zone of specialized smooth muscle in the distal esophagus just rostral to the esophagogastric mucosal junction, normally lies at the point where the diaphragm muscle abuts the esophagus. Intraluminal manometry detects the LES as a zone of raised resting pressure, caused by a stable tonic contraction of the circular muscle layer. This area of tonic contraction, evident in the elevated resting pressure, is very important because a reduction in this pressure is associated with GERD, which is one of the most common of all pathologic conditions. In Fig. 2.2B, a normal color contour of the LES is seen. It appears as a horizontal band of color indicating pressure greater than intragastric or intraesophageal pressure. It migrates up and down with respiration. This occurs as a result of the diaphragm movement. During inspiration the diaphragm contracts and the contour moves down. With expiration the diapharagm relaxes and the contour moves up. The accompanying variations in intraabdominal and intrathoracic pressures are clearly seen (Fig. 2.2B).

Figure 2.3 shows the LES relaxation associated with a swallow. LES relaxation produces a color change to approximate that of gastric basal pressure. This allows the bolus to pass through ahead of esophageal peristalsis. What is also evident is that the LES contracts vigorously upon arrival of the peristaltic contraction.

---

record pressure data from the pharynx, UES, esophagus, LES, and proximal stomach. Alterations in intraesophageal pressure generated by respiration produce cyclical variations in color indicating lower pressure during inspiration and higher pressure during expiration. Resting UES and LES pressures are seen as horizontal bands of color that are several centimeters wide. The pressure generated in each is greater than in the adjacent pharynx, esophagus, or stomach. Two structures, the LES and the diaphragm, combine to generate a high-pressure zone (HPZ) in the region of the gastroesophageal (GE) junction. This pressure varies cyclically in position and amplitude. During inspiration, the HPZ displaces toward the stomach and increases in amplitude (*). These changes are caused by diaphragmatic contraction. Expiration is associated with movement of the HPZ toward the esophagus and a diminution in pressure. Pressure recorded at the HPZ during expiration is thought to be characteristic of resting LES pressure (LESP), and by convention is reported as such. Normal resting LESP recorded by HRM ranges from 10 to 35 mmHg. Location of the diaphragm can also be determined by identifying the pressure inversion point (PIP). The PIP is the location along the recording segment at which cyclical pressure changes produced by respiration change in phase by 180 degrees. This occurs because pressure in the chest decreases with inspiration and increases with expiration, while in the abdomen the opposite occurs. Here, the respiratory inversion occurs across the HPZ, indicating that the LES and diaphragm are in approximately the same location.

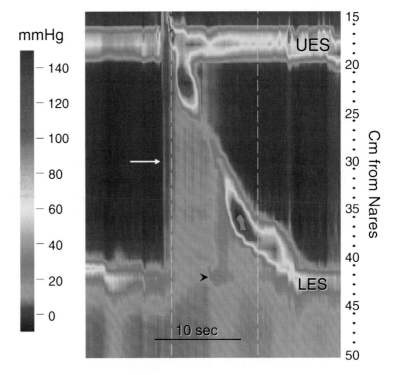

Fig. 2.3. Effect of diaphragmatic contraction on intrabolus pressure. This high-resolution color contour of a normal peristaltic sequence and LES relaxation depicts the effect of diaphragmatic contraction on intrabolus pressure. The *white arrow* indicates the intrabolus pressure resulting from a WS. The intrabolus pressure is seen as a simultaneous change in hue to a lighter blue, indicating a small increase in pressure. The *arrowhead* points to an increase in pressure produced by diaphragmatic contraction during inspiration. This contraction is associated temporally with a band of green color that runs vertically from the GE junction to the peristaltic sequence. This color change indicates a rise in intrabolus pressure. It likely occurs because diaphragmatic contraction presents a barrier to bolus clearance. When the diaphragm relaxes intrabolus pressure drops.

The LES is much more reliably tracked in HRM than it is in conventional manometry. One major problem with the conventional manometric techniques is that they may not track axial LES movements. These techniques rely on a small number of widely spaced sensors straddling the LES. A drop in pressure may represent either relaxation of the LES or esophageal shortening that puts the LES out of the range of a sensor. Thus, older manometric techniques may not recognize failed LES relaxation.

2.1.5. Normal Bolus Pressure

Intrabolus pressure, the pressure generated in the liquid bolus by the muscular contraction behind it, can be difficult to appreciate with older techniques (Fig.1.4A) unless the pressure is very pronounced. Fig. 2.3 depicts this pressurization on a high-resolution color contour.

2.1.6. Peristalsis

Figures 1.4F, 2.1 and 2.3 all depict high-resolution color contours of normal primary esophageal peristaltic sequences produced by water swallows. The warmer colors reveal the migrating pressure wave toward the LES. The colors demonstrate how uniform and complete the sequence is. There are no gaps in the migrating event besides the attenuation in the transition zone mentioned above.

2.1.7. Gastric Pressures

High-resolution manometry clearly demonstrates changes in intragastric pressure. Conventional manometry usually can show them only with deep inspiration, but not during the shallow breathing usual in the resting state. On the other hand, HRM reveals the excursions in intragastric pressure during breathing (Fig. 2.2B).

2.2. Abnormal High-Resolution Esophageal Manometry

Abnormal motor functions characteristic of specific clinical disorders often appear as patterns made by the color contour, so diagnosis usually involves pattern recognition.

2.2.1. Achalasia

The features of achalasia identified by conventional manometry include aperistalsis in the smooth muscle esophagus and failed or incomplete LES relaxation. However, HRM provides many more details. Table 2.2 lists these features of achalasia that are more easily seen with HRM color contours.

The conventional manometry in figure 2.4A is from a patient with achalasia, It reveals incomplete LES relaxation and failure of peristalsis with a swallow. The corresponding HRM contour is seen in Fig. 2.4B . The LES relaxation is clearly impaired, and isobaric pressure waves are easily seen. However, with the HRM contour we are now able to see new details in achalasia. In some cases there are profound changes in the LES location. The LES appears to rise, suggesting esophageal shortening (Fig. 2.4 and 2.6). In some cases, as in Fig. 2.5 , the shortening may be of considerable magnitude. In this example, it was 7 to 8 cm. Moreover, the shortening is accompanied by a significant, greater than 50 mmHg, increase in pressure throughout the esophageal body. Such changes are not as conspicuous with conventional manometry.

High-resolution manometry also clearly reveals two other phenomena in achalasia. The first is the total esophageal pressurization that occurs cyclically, as in Figures 2.6, 2.7, and 2.8 . The second is rhythmic UES contractions at rest, that

Table 2.2. Characteristics of achalasia with high-resolution manometry.

1. Incomplete LES relaxation
2. Absence of peristalsis in the esophagus
3. Esophageal pressurization during wet swallows
4. Persistent pressurization of esophagus between wet swallows (isobaric pressure waves)
5. Esophageal shortening (sometimes dramatic)
6. Depressurization of esophagus with UES relaxation

UES, upper esophageal sphincter.

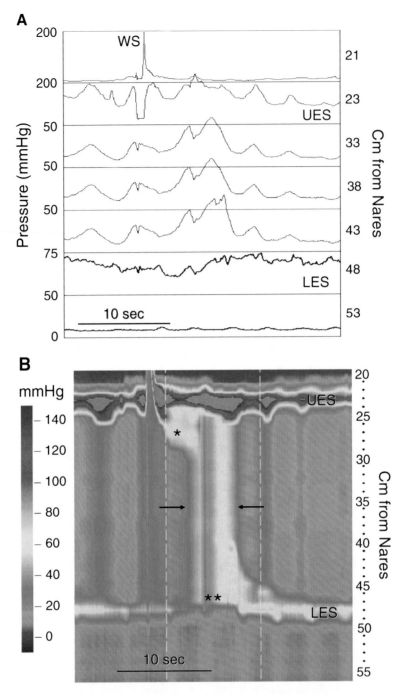

Fig. 2.4. Conventional manometry and high-resolution color contour in achalasia. (A) A manometry displayed in line mode as a conventional manometry demonstrates typical features of achalasia. Instead of peristalsis, a WS produces simultaneous, repetitive pressure waves in the smooth muscle esophagus that appear nearly identical from one channel to the next. These are called isobaric pressure waves, and they occur because the esophagus is behaving as a common cavity. Also, the LES does not relax completely. (B) The same pressure data are displayed as a high-resolution color contour. The striated muscle esophagus generates a peristaltic pressure wave (*), but the diagonal band of color characteristic of smooth muscle peristalsis is not present. Instead, there are vertical bands of color that are indicative of simultaneous, isobaric pressure waves (between *arrows*). The color band depicting resting LES pressure changes little, and does not approximate the color portraying intragastric pressure following the WS. This indicates failed or incomplete LES relaxation, a diagnostic feature of achalasia. The LES moves cephalad a few centimeters, indicating esophageal shortening (**).

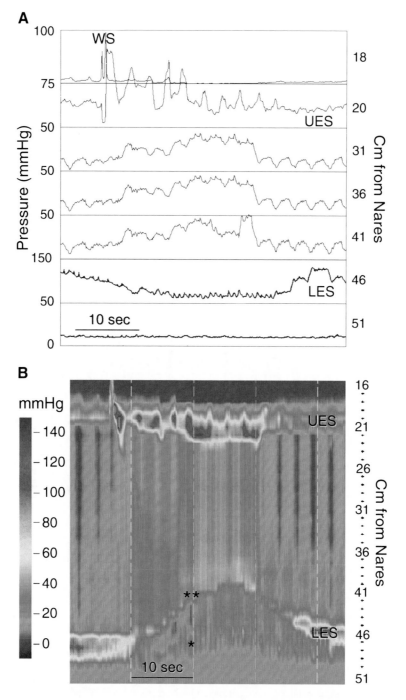

Fig. 2.5. Achalasia: esophageal shortening and hiatus hernia. (A) In this high-resolution manometry displayed in line mode, a WS produces simultaneous, isobaric pressure waves in the esophagus, and what appears to be a prolonged LES (>30 seconds) relaxation recorded by a 6-cm-long eSleeve centered on the LES. The genesis of this unusual recording is easily ascertained in the HRM color contour from the same data (B). The WS initiates a marked (7 to 8 cm) cephalad movement of the LES, which is associated with contraction of the UES and a rise in intraesophageal pressure. The LES (**) is pulled above the diaphragm (*) to produce a hiatus hernia. The position of the diaphragm coincides with the pressure inversion point—the location along the recording segment at which cyclical pressure changes produced by respiration change in phase by 180 degrees (see Fig. 2.2). The apparent LES relaxation in A is an artifact of profound esophageal shortening that pulls the LES cephalad to all of the eSleeve sensors. Therefore, the conventional line manometry may be misread as showing LES relaxation.

S. Jee; M. Pimentel; E. Soffer; JL. Conklin: A High-Resolution View of Achalasia, J Clin Gastroenterol volume 00, Number 00, December 18, 2008 PUBLISHED AHEAD OF PRINT.

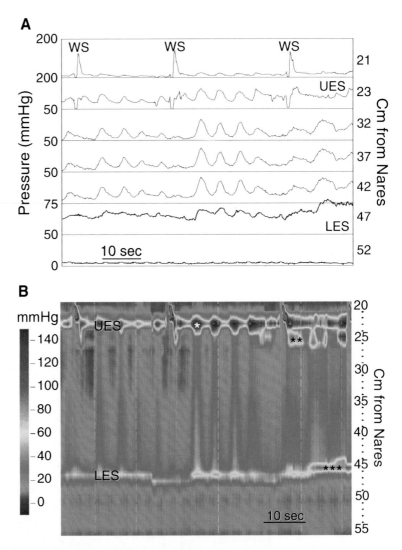

Fig. 2.6. Esophageal motor responses to repeated WSs in achalasia. (A) The high-resolution manometry displayed in line mode demonstrates typical features of achalasia: repetitive isobaric pressure waves induced by WS and incomplete LES relaxation. The same pressure data displayed as a high-resolution color contour (B) reveal features of achalasia not readily apparent with conventional manometry. In this case, resting intraesophageal pressure increases and the esophagus shortens (***). The repetitive, isobaric pressure waves generated by WSs are associated temporally with contraction of the UES (*). As more swallows are taken, more striated esophageal muscle is recruited in the contractile process (**), and these contractile activities increase in intensity and duration.

S. Jee; M. Pimentel; E. Soffer; JL. Conklin: A High-Resolution View of Achalasia, J Clin Gastroenterol volume 00, Number 00, December 18, 2008 PUBLISHED AHEAD OF PRINT.

correspond temporally with the cyclical, isobaric pressure waves in the esophageal body (Figs 2.6, 2.7 and 2.8). Some would argue that these oscillations are respiratory, but the HRM contour (Fig 2.7B) shows that diaphragmatic contractions do not occur in concert with oscillations in intraesophageal pressure.

Records from another case of achalasia (Fig. 2.8) show how depressurization of the esophagus by an esophageal belch alters the oscillatory behavior characteristic of achalasia. Notice that transient opening of the UES depres-

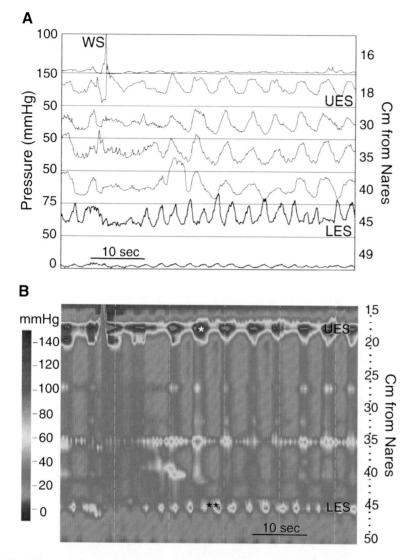

Fig. 2.7. Achalasia: high-resolution manometry demonstrating the relationship between repetitive pressure waves and respiration. (A) The high-resolution manometry displayed in line mode demonstrates prominent, repetitive, simultaneous, isobaric pressure waves characteristic of achalasia. The same pressure data displayed as a high-resolution color contour (B) reveal features not readily apparent with conventional manometry. The repetitive, isobaric pressure waves in the esophagus are associated with contraction of the UES and striated muscle esophagus (*). One possible interpretation of these pressure waves is that they result from respiration. In fact, pressure transients associated with diaphragmatic contraction during respiration (**) occur at a rate different from the esophageal pressure waves. This indicates that the repetitive esophageal pressure waves are not caused by respiration.

surizes the esophagus and shuts off oscillations in esophageal pressure until another wet swallow occured. The "esophageal belch" is relatively common in achalasia.

Variant forms of achalasia best described as "vigorous achalasia" are seen in Figure 2.9 - 2.11. In all cases there are high amplitude pressure waves that do not propagate and failed or incomplete LES relaxation. In one case there is retrograde peristalsis (Fig. 2.11).

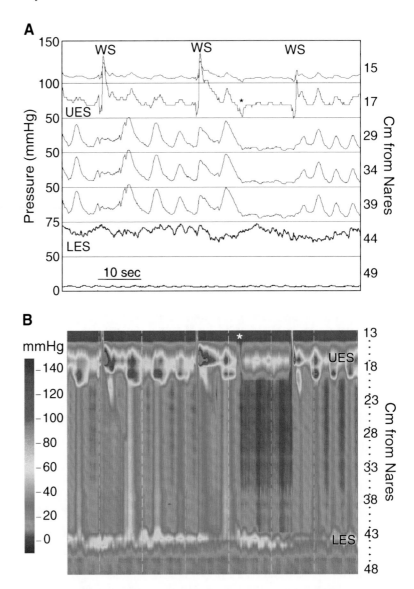

Fig. 2.8. Achalasia: the esophageal belch. (A) This high-resolution manometry displayed in line mode shows typical features of achalasia. After the second WS, repetitive isobaric pressure waves cease until the next WS. The likely mechanism by which this occurs is easily seen in the HRM color contour. There is transient relaxation of the UES (*) that allows venting of the esophagus. This lowers resting intraesophageal pressure and interrupts generation of repetitive, isobaric pressure waves until more water is swallowed. This phenomenon is not easily seen in the conventional recording because the technique does not allow simultaneous recording from the UES and entire smooth muscle segment. In addition, conventional manometry does not reliably record UES motor function.

S. Jee; M. Pimentel; E. Soffer; JL. Conklin: A High-Resolution View of Achalasia, J Clin Gastroenterol volume 00, Number 00, December 18, 2008 PUBLISHED AHEAD OF PRINT.

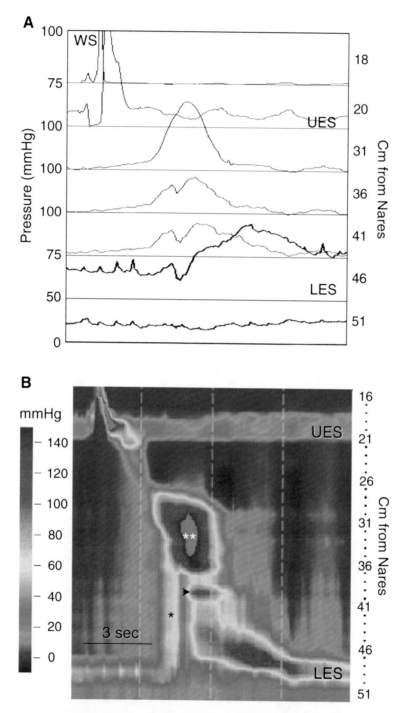

Fig. 2.9. Achalasia with bolus entrapment. (A) This high-resolution manometry displayed in line mode shows a WS that produces simultaneous pressure waves at all three recording sites in the esophagus. There is failure of LES relaxation. The morphology of the top pressure wave (31 cm) differs from that of the lower two pressure waves (36 and 41 cm), suggesting that they arise from different processes. (B) The HRM color contour proves this to be the case, and provides more information about this motor event. There is peristalsis over a short segment of the smooth muscle esophagus that ends in a powerful contraction of the mid-esophagus (**). The pink color indicates a pressure that is out of range, >150 mmHg. This strong contraction pressurizes the bolus (*) against a closed LES. There is also a smaller segmental contraction (*arrowhead*) that is essentially impossible to see on the line mode tracing. The HRM contour also reveals a low resting UES pressure, in the range of 20 mmHg.

A common reason for conducting manometry in achalasia is to evaluate patients who remain symptomatic after Heller myotomy. The HRM color contour helps identify the adequacy of a myotomy. A low resting LES pressure signifies an adequate myotomy (Fig. 2.13), while a normal or high resting pressure indicates an inadequate myotomy (Fig 2.14). The isobaric lines help show that the LES resting pressure is greater than 20 mmHg. Notice that the esophagus still fails to produce peristalsis, even when the myotomy is successful Fig. 2.13.

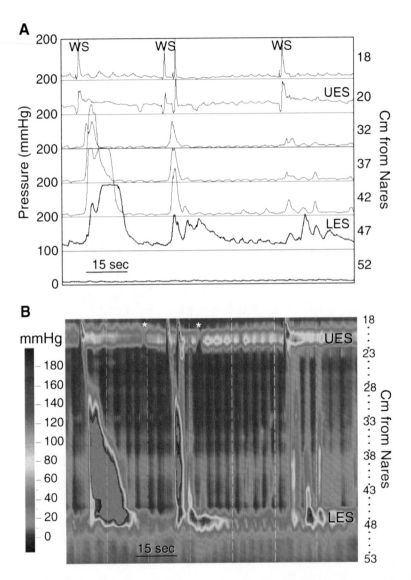

Fig. 2.10. Vigorous achalasia. (A) In this high-resolution manometry displayed in line mode, WSs produce simultaneous pressure waves that take quite different configurations. The first has pressures >200 mmHg and a prolonged duration in the distal esophagus. The second has a shorter duration but high amplitude. Following the third WS, there is a lower amplitude simultaneous pressure wave. (B) The HRM color contour demonstrates these findings but accentuates several others: there are incomplete or failed LES relaxations, transient relaxations of the UES (*), and repetitive simultaneous pressure waves in the distal esophagus following the third WS.

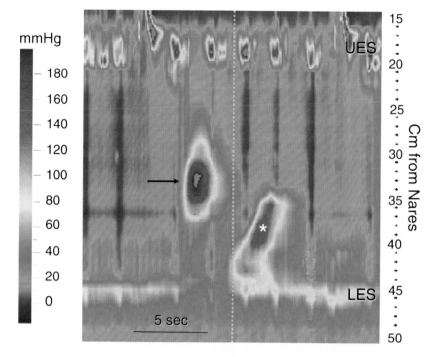

Fig. 2.11. Retrograde peristalsis and incomplete LES relaxation. A WS produces an isolated high-amplitude (>200 mmHg) pressure wave in the mid-esophagus (*arrow*) that is followed by a retrograde peristaltic sequence in the distal esophagus (*). Relaxation of the LES is incomplete and delayed in onset. This contour likely represents a variant of achalasia.

Incomplete relaxation can be observed not just in achalasia. It can be seen as an isolated finding in patients with normal peristalsis (Fig. 2.15), a distal esophageal stricture, or a Nissen fundoplication (Fig. 2.38).

2.2.2. Diffuse Esophageal Spasm

Diffuse esophageal spasm is defined broadly as uncoordinated motor activity in the smooth muscle esophagus. To make the diagnois there must be simultaneous pressure waves associated with >10%, but <100% of wet swallows. The mean amplitude of simultaneous pressure waves must be >30mmHg. Other features of spasm include; spontaneous contractions, repetitive contractions, multipeaked contractions and some normal peristalsis (Figs.2.16 and 2.17). The color contour suggests that spasm maybe segmental. For example, in Figure 2.16C,D there is normal peristalsis in the proximal esophagus, but over a roughly 9-cm segment of the mid-esophagus.
This segmental spasm could easily be missed with conventional manometry. The patient also had simultaneous, high-amplitude and prolonged pressure waves (Figs. 2.16A,B), high-amplude peristalsis and normal amplitude simultaneous pressure waves (Fig. 2.16E,F). An example of the repetitive smooth mucle contractile activity that might be seen in spasm is shown in figure 2.17. Notice that the multipeaked pressure waves seen with conventional manometry are actually temporally and spatially distinct from one another, an observation that is not obvious on the conventional manometry.

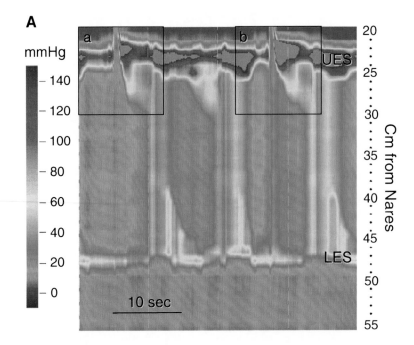

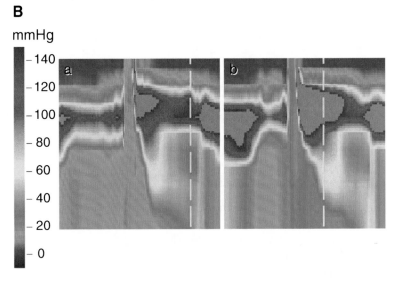

Fig. 2.12. Residual UES pressure in achalasia. (A) This HRM color contour of two WSs in achalasia demonstrates failure of peristalsis and LES relaxation. The boxes (a and b) demarcate areas of the proximal esophagus around UES opening. The areas enclosed by the boxes are magnified to detail the UES in B. In both cases the color indicating pressure at the location of the open UES approximates that in the proximal esophagus. This means that residual UES pressure reflects proximal esophageal pressure at the time of UES opening. Thus, the elevated residual UES pressure reported in achalasia is a function of intraesophageal pressure rather than dysfunction of the UES.

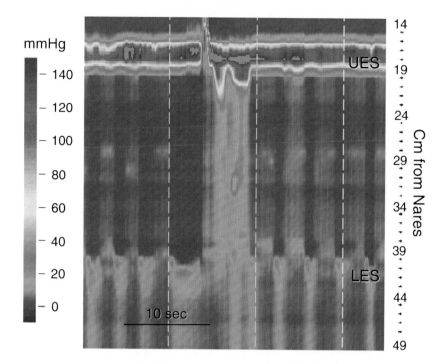

Fig. 2.13. Successfully treated achalasia. This HRM color contour is from a patient after Heller myotomy. Peristalsis is present in the striated muscle esophagus, but not in the smooth muscle segment. Resting LES pressure is low (<10 mmHg), indicating a successful myotomy.

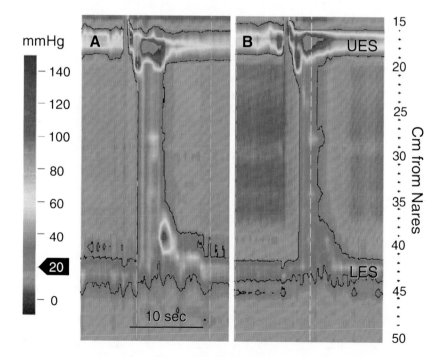

Fig. 2.14. Failed achalasia treatment. These HRM color contours are from a patient with achalasia before (A) and after (B) Heller myotomy. In both cases, there is failure of LES relaxation, and simultaneous isobaric pressure waves in the esophageal body. The black lines bordering the color contours are isobaric pressure lines generated by the computer to indicate when and where the pressure is 20 mmHg. Inside these lines the pressure is >20 mmHg and outside the lines it is <20 mmHg. (B) After myotomy, resting LES pressure remains >20 mmHg, indicating that the myotomy is incomplete.

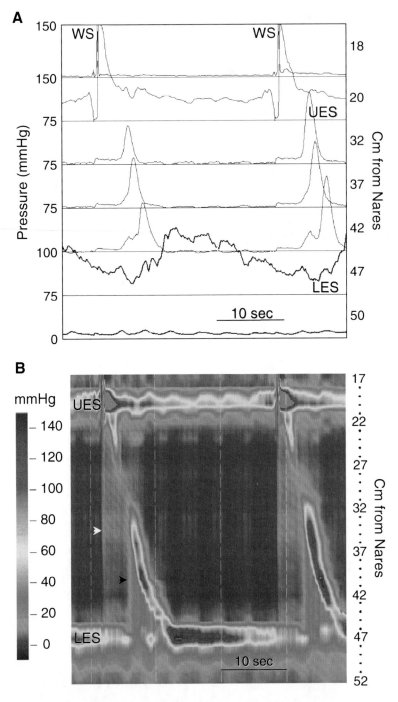

Fig. 2.15. Incomplete LES relaxation. (A) A recording of two WSs from a patient complaining of dysphagia is displayed in line mode as a conventional manometry. There is normal peristalsis in the striated and smooth muscle segments of the esophagus. The LES appears to have a high resting pressure, but it does relax. (B) The HRM color contour of these same swallows. While there is normal esophageal motor function, the LES behaves abnormally. The LES should relax shortly after opening of the UES and approximate the intragastric pressure (see Figs. 1.4F and 2.3). In this HRM contour LES relaxation is delayed and its pressure remains well above intragastric pressure throughout most of the time it should be relaxed. This is seen as a persistence of yellow and green colors at the location of the LES after UES opening. Also notice what happens to intrabolus pressure as the peristaltic sequence progresses. There is an initial small rise in intraesophageal pressure when the bolus is swallowed (*white arrowhead*). Peristalsis in the smooth muscle esophagus is associated with a significant rise in intrabolus pressure (*black arrowhead*). This indicates that the esophagus is compressing the bolus against a closed GE junction.

Table 2.3. Issues with high-resolution manometry in diagnosing esophageal spasm.

Spasm and high-resolution manometry (HRM):

1. May have to avoid the term *diffuse* when referring to spasm
2. Often find isolated spasm in a segment of the esophagus (is this spasm also?)
3. Rarely diffuse or involving the whole esophagus
4. Multiphasic contractions are commonly repetitive or retrograde contractions
5. HRM seems to identify more cases of spasm due to close spacing of channels

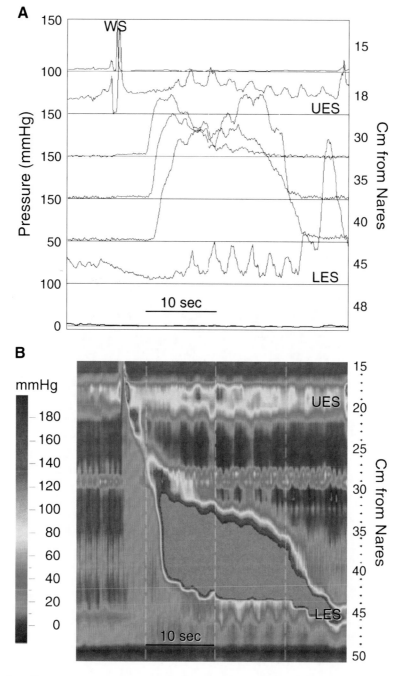

Fig. 2.16. (continued)

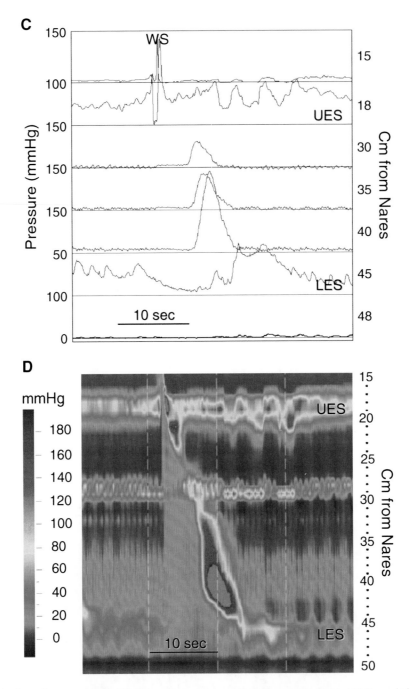

Fig. 2.16. Esophageal spasm. (A–F) All of these recordings are from the same subject. (A) Recorded in line mode, a WS generates a high-amplitude, long-duration pressure wave that propagates very rapidly. (B) The HRM contour plot of the same swallow reveals normal peristalsis in the proximal esophagus and normal LES relaxation with residual LES pressure approximating intragastric pressure. Onset of the high-amplitude, long-duration pressure wave is essentially simultaneous over several centimeters of the distal esophagus. This is not easily appreciated with the conventional line tracing. The pink color indicates that the pressure is >200 mmHg. In fact, the pressure is over 500 mmHg. (C) A WS produces normal LES relaxation and a simultaneous pressure wave in

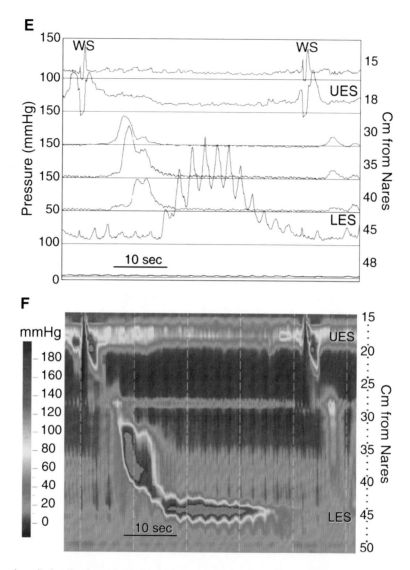

Fig. 2.16. (continued) the distal esophagus that is of high amplitude. (D) The HRM color contour generated from the same swallow. Line (E) and HRM (F) contour plots from two WSs are compared. The first swallow generates a high-amplitude pressure wave that is peristaltic, and normal LES relaxation that is followed by a marked rebound rise in LES pressure (>200 mmHg). The second produces a much weaker simultaneous pressure wave in the smooth muscle esophagus. The esophageal motor abnormalities seen in this subject are what might be expected in esophageal spasm.

The use of HRM color contours is likely to provide details that will help reclassify what are likely to be a several motor disorders that are now called "spasm." Sme of the issues raised using HRM to diagnose spasm are presented in table 2.3.

2.2.3. Nutcracker Esophagus

While the so-called nutcracker esophagus is readily identifiable by both conventional (Fig. 2.18A) and high-resolution manometry (Fig. 2.18B), it is easily recognizable in color high-resolution (Fig. 2.18B). The color scheme of the HRM can provide this diagnosis at a glance.

2.2.4. Hiatal Hernia

High-resolution manometry reliably identifies hiatal herniation (provided it is present at the time of recording). Fig. 2.19 shows high-resolution color contour of a large (8 cm) hiatal hernia. Notice the two pressure zones of elevated resting pressure (one at 41 cm, the other at 49 cm) (Fig. 2.19A). The peristaltic sequence travels down to the zone at 41 cm, indicating that this is the LES. In further confirmation of this, the diaphragm as identified by the PIP at 49 cm. Recall the PIP is the location at which pressure changesproduced by respiration go out of phase by 180 degrees (Fig. 2.2). This means the gastric segment between 42 and 49 cm lies in the thoracic cavity. As described in the figure legend, Fig. 2.19B shows a method of identifying the diaphragm. HRM is particularly useful in cases of small hiatal hernia, as shown in Figs. 2.20 and 2.21.

2.2.5. Gastroesophageal Reflux Disease and Lower Esophageal Sphincter

Low resting pressure in the LES strongly favors the development of GERD. The degree of LES dysfunction becomes clear with the use of color in manometric records. Fig. 2.20 and 2.21 demonstrate examples; in this casees, little or no resting pressure can be seen in the LES. In addition, there is a small hiatal hernia in each.

2.2.6. Scleroderma

Scleroderma is classically associated with motor disturbances of the esophagus. As in nutcracker esophagus, the findings in scleroderma esophagus are readily apparent. Typically, scleroderma involves a neuropathic and later myopathic dysfunction of gastrointestinal smooth muscle. This typically results in the observation of preserved upper esophageal peristalsis and absent or weak distal peristalsis. In addition, the LES pressure is low or negligible. Fig. 2.23 is a good example of this. Notice the fully intact resting UES pressure and opening. Other features characteristic of scleroderma, such as the lack of peristalsis and low LES resting pressure, are also easy to identify.

2.2.7. Ineffective Esophageal Motility

Ineffective esophageal motor dysfunction refers to a collection of findings or values in manometry of the esophagus that are outside the normal range. Very little is known about the physiologic cause or significance of these findings except that they reduce the effectiveness of bolus transit through the esophagus. One example of this is low-amplitude esophageal peristalsis. Fig. 2.24A demonstrates this in conventional format. The corresponding high-resolution format is shown in Fig. 2.24b. In this image, the color shows the force of peristaltic contractions to be very low. Isobaric lines can add clarity to such

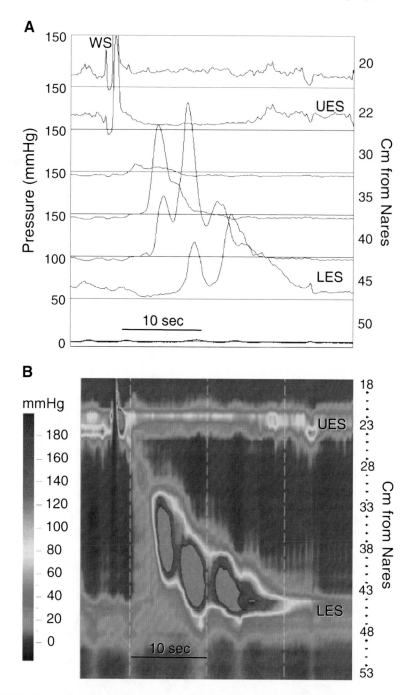

Fig. 2.17. Multiphasic esophageal pressure waves. (A) In this manometry displayed in line mode to simulate a conventional manometry tracing, a WS produces repetitive, high-amplitude pressure waves in the distal esophagus, 5 cm above the LES. (B) A HRM color contour generated from the same swallow provides more spatial and temporal information regarding this phenomenon. There are actually three esophageal contractions that are temporally and spatially distinct from one another. In the line mode they look like a single multiphasic contraction. The pink color indicates pressures >200 mmHg. Together, this chain of contractile activity produces a peristalsis sequence.

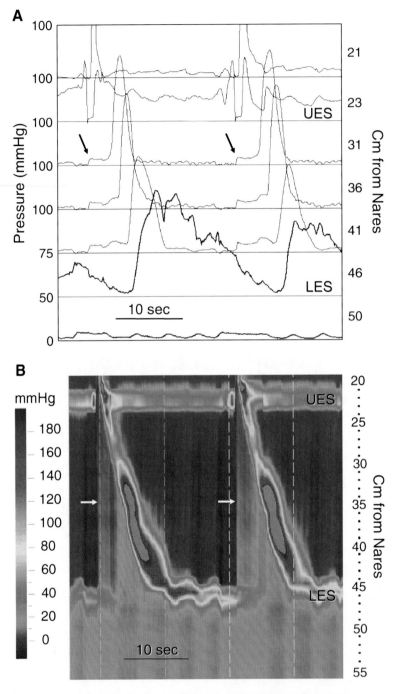

Fig. 2.18. Nutcracker or hypertensive peristalsis. A manometry displayed in line mode to simulate a conventional tracing (A) and an HRM color contour (B) from a subject with hypertensive peristalsis are compared. Wet swallows (WSs) produce very high-amplitude peristaltic sequences. There is also an obvious bolus pressure ahead of the peristaltic pressure waves (*arrows* in both A and B). In the conventional recording this is seen as a step up in pressure to a plateau ahead of the peristaltic pressure wave. In the HRM contour, it is seen as a simultaneous shift to a lighter blue (higher pressure) coinciding with opening of the UES, and is bounded on the right by the peristaltic pressure wave. Following passage of the peristaltic wave, the color returns to a darker blue, indicating a drop in intraesophageal pressure and clearance of the bolus.

A

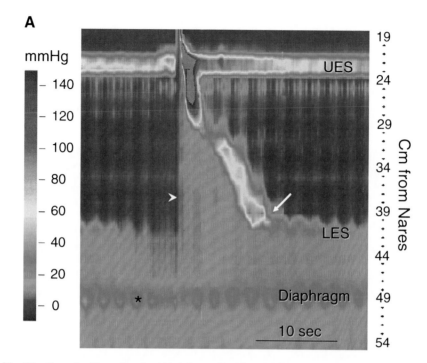

Fig. 2.19. Identification of a hiatus hernia. (A) A large (7 to 8 cm) hiatus hernia is identified in this HRM color contour. There are two zones of high pressure in proximity to the gastroesophageal junction. One appears as a horizontal band of green color about 49 cm from the nares. This band of color coincides with the pressure inversion point (PIP) (*) that defines the location of the diaphragm (see Fig. 2.2). The PIP is the point above which inspiration decreases intrathoracic pressure (change to a darker blue), and below which it increases intraabdominal pressure (change to a lighter blue). This is the pattern of pressure change seen above and below the *asterisk*. The second zone of high pressure arises as a horizontal band of green color at the distal extent of the peristaltic pressure wave (*arrow*), roughly 41 cm from the nares. Notice that when the peristaltic pressure wave arrives at the LES, the color contour produces an obtuse angle (*arrow*). This is a characteristic feature that helps identify the LES location. An intraesophageal bolus pressure is easily seen ahead of the peristaltic pressure wave (*arrowhead*). The bolus pressure is transmitted across the GE junction into the hernia, but not across the diaphragm. Following passage of the peristaltic wave, the color indicating intraesophageal pressure returns to a darker blue, indicating a drop in intraesophageal pressure and clearance of the bolus. Also, the hernia appears to pressurize as the peristaltic wave progresses toward the GE junction. In fact, at the end of the peristaltic sequence pressure in the hernia is greater than in the esophagus or remainder of the stomach. (B) A software tool that aids in identifying the diaphragm (PIP) is demonstrated. This HRM color contour plot comes from the same study as in A. At the bottom of the figure, there are three horizontal, colored lines that are 1 cm apart: blue at 47 cm, red at 48 cm, and green at 49 cm from the nares. The box near the middle of the contour also displays three colored lines. These lines show the pressures recorded at the positions of their corresponding colored lines at 47, 48, and 49 cm from the nares. The three colored lines at the bottom can be moved up and down as a unit. They are positioned here to identify the location of the diaphragm (PIP). The *arrowhead* points to the changes in presswure produced by inspiration. Notice that with inspiration the blue line indicates a drop in pressure and the green line indicates a rise in pressure. This means that the blue line (47 cm) is above the diaphragm and the green line (49 cm) is below the diaphragm. The diaphragm (PIP) is therefore between 47 and 49 cm from the nares. When the red line is located at the diaphragm, the waveform becomes flat or biphasic.

images. These are the black lines seen in the image. Any pressures within these black outlined areas are above 30 mmHg. Notice that most of the peristalsis does not achieve this in the first swallow; the second swallow never achieves the necessary propulsive pressure for effective bolus transfer (Fig. 2.24).

B

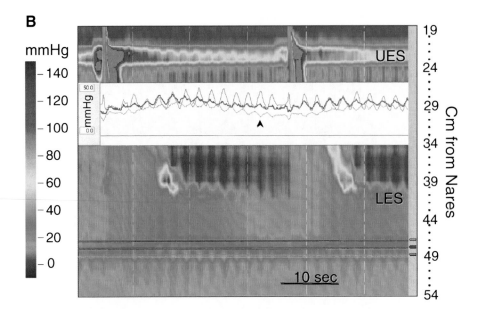

Fig. 2.19. (continued)

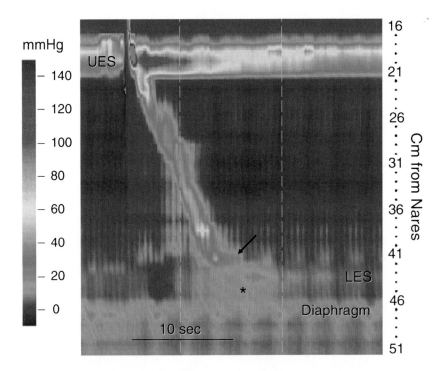

Fig. 2.20. Hypotensive LES and small hiatus hernia. In this HRM color contour, the UES and body of the esophagus function normally. The LES is located 42 to 43 cm from the nares, and is very weak and nearly indistinguishable from intragastric pressure. Looking for the obtuse angle made by the peristaltic pressure wave and LES (*arrow*) helps in its identification. The diaphragm is located 47 to 48 cm from the nares. Notice that as in the previous figure the hernia appears to be transiently and subtly pressurized by the peristaltic sequence (*).

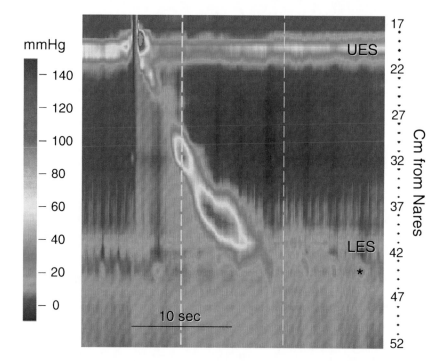

Fig. 2.21. Hypotensive LES and incipient hiatus hernia. In this HRM color contour the UES and body of the esophagus function normally. The LES is hypotensive, but visible as a region of elevated pressure just above the diaphragm (*).

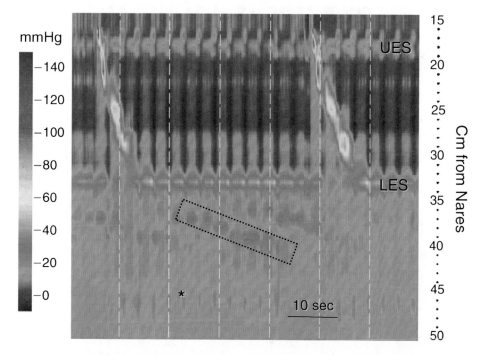

Fig. 2.22. Large hiatus hernia and hypotensive UES. This HRM color contour is from a patient with much of the stomach herniated into the chest. Notice that resting UES pressure is quite low, in the range of 20 mmHg. Esophageal and LES motor function appear normal, but the esophagus is short, measuring about 15 cm in length. In addition, the respiratory PIP is not located at the GE junction. Careful inspection of the contour plot reveals that the PIP (*) is present about 46 cm from the nares, indicating that there is a very large, approximately 13 cm, hiatus hernia. There is also a cyclical alteration in pressure within the hernia that has a periodicity of about 20 seconds, and appears to propagate antegrade; one such pressure wave is seen in the diagonal box. These are the characteristics of gastric antral contractions.

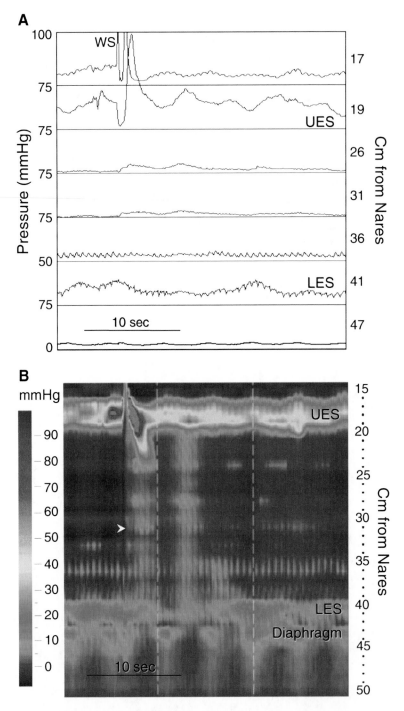

Fig. 2.23. Scleroderma. (A) This is a high-resolution manometry from a patient with scleroderma displayed in line mode. A WS generates normal relaxation of the UES, but no esophageal peristalsis. It is difficult to determine if there is relaxation of the LES. If we did not know that this recording was from a person with scleroderma, it would not be easy to distinguish from achalasia. (B) In the HRM color contour from the same WS we see normal UES resting pressure and relaxation, and normal peristalsis in the striated muscle esophagus. There is aperistalsis of the smooth muscle esophagus. At the GE junction there is a small hiatus hernia, and the LES relaxes appropriately. Notice that the WS generates a bolus pressure (*arrowhead*) seen as a simultaneous shift to a lighter blue (higher pressure) coinciding with opening of the UES. In the absence of a peristaltic pressure wave the lighter blue color only slowly returns toward the darker blue seen in the empty esophagus. This indicates that the bolus was not cleared from the esophagus.

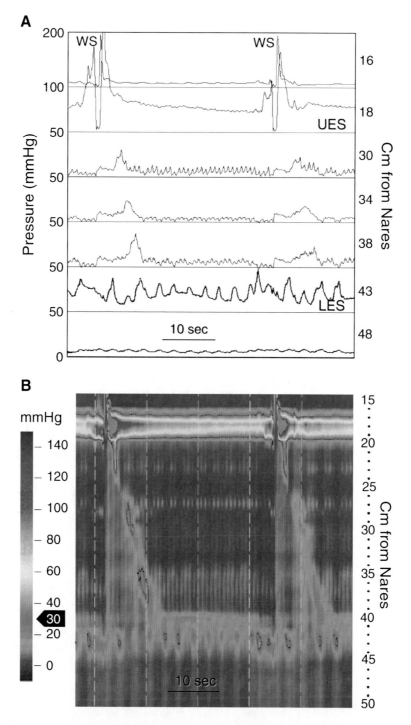

Fig. 2.24. Ineffective esophageal motility. (A) A recording of two WSs displayed to simulate a conventional manometric tracing. There is peristalsis in the smooth muscle esophagus, but its amplitude appears low. (B) In the HRM color contour from the same wet swallows, isobaric contour lines (black lines) set at 30 mmHg were used to determine if and when peristaltic pressures dropped below 30 mmHg; pressures inside the isobaric lines are >30 mmHg. Thirty millimeters of mercury was chosen because it is the current convention for defining ineffective esophageal peristalsis. The first WS produced a peristaltic pressure wave that was above 30 mmHg over two short segments of the smooth muscle esophagus, and the second WS generated a peristaltic pressure wave below 30 mmHg along the entire smooth muscle segment. Also note that there is a hypotensive LES.

2.2.8. Cricopharyngeal Bar

The UES composed of the inferior pharyngeal constrictor, cricopharyneus and cricoid cartilage. Cricopharyngeal bar is a radiographic term to describe a thickened cricopharyngeus that indents the lumen at the pharyngoesophageal junction on barium swallow. The muscle is fibrosed, so the UES does not open easily with swallowing. It typically produces dysphagia. Until the advent of HRM, technical difficulties made it impossble to reliably evaluate the UES with manometry. When looking at the UES of this patient with dysphagia and a radiographically documented cricopharyngeal bar (Fig 2.26), there is a yellow color defect at the UES and pharynx during a swallow. The color should normally be close to isobaric with the esophagus when the UES opens. In this case, the yellow color suggests an elevated pharyngeal bolus pressure above a functional or mechanical obstruction. Figure 2.26B shows this feature in greater detail.

2.2.9. Other Esophageal Observations with High-Resolution Manometry

The examples shown above are common HRM findings in the esophagus. The next series of images depict less common cases of esophageal diseases. The interpretation of these images requires a thorough understanding of HRM and

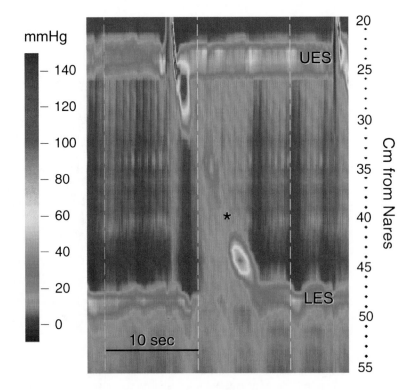

Fig. 2.25. Ineffective esophageal motility. This HRM color contour demonstrates normal function of the UES, striated muscle esophagus, and LES. There is no hiatus hernia. There is dropout of the peristaltic sequence in the middle of the smooth muscle segment (*).

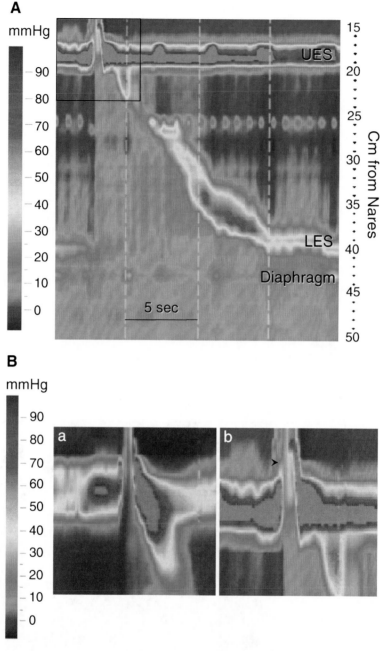

Fig. 2.26. Cricopharyngeal bar. (A) An HRM color contour demonstrating a WS from a patient with a cricopharyngeal bar. Peristalsis is normal in the striated and smooth muscle segments of the esophagus. There is a 2- to 3-cm hiatus hernia, and the LES relaxes appropriately. Note the area circumscribed by the box at the upper left corner of the figure. (B) This area (b) and a similar area from a normal study (a) are expanded. Normally, during UES opening residual UES pressure drops to approximate intraesophageal pressure. This is seen in as a change in color to the blue hues denoting intraesophageal pressures below the UES (a). Residual UES pressure does not drop to approximate intraesophageal pressure in this patient with a cricopharyngeal bar (b). In addition, pressure in the pharynx above the UES is elevated (*arrowhead*) ahead of the pharyngeal peristaltic sequence. This indicates an elevated bolus pressure that suggests functional obstruction at the level of the UES. The HRM color contour's ability to easily identify elevated pharyngeal and residual UES pressures is a significant advantage over conventional manometric techniques.

its power in detecting specific events in the esophagus. In most cases, HRM identified features that assist in the diagnosis and management of the patient that would have been very difficult to detect with conventional manometry.

Fig. 2.27 is an HRM contour from a patient with polymyositis. In this case, the patient suffered with dysphagia. The HRM in this image shows a number of abnormalities. There is a global disturbance of motor function. The UES resting pressure is greatly reduced. The LES resting pressure was normal. Additionally, the esophagus produced no effective peristaltic pressures.

Fig. 2.28 is another case of dysphagia. This time the patient had a known history of myasthenia gravis. While the classic features of gradually diminishing motor activity were not seen, a global striated motor disturbance was seen with the LES pressure remaining intact.

The patient in Fig. 2.29 had laryngeal cancer and subsequent radiation therapy some years prior to this manometric recording. This image shows the destructive effects of this previous radiation on the operation of the UES and upper esophageal motor activity. While the test cannot discriminate neurologic from myopathic causes, the result is clearly abnormal and accounts for profound symptoms of oropharyngeal and upper esophageal dysphagia. Notice the near absence of pharyngeal contractile response with swallows. The distal esophageal motor events are still triggered to occur after a swallow, indicating that the muscle and intramural nerves are functional to drive the distal esophageal body, outside of the field of radiation.

Fig. 2.30 and 2.37 show examples of transient LES relaxation. HRM clearly shows the typical sequence of events that would be very difficult to interpret

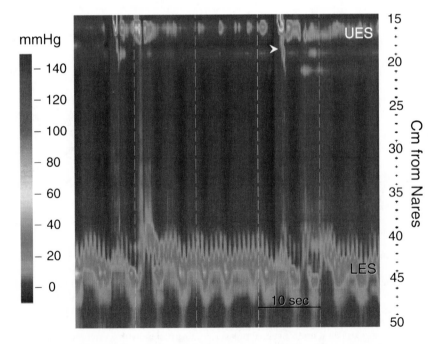

Fig. 2.27. Failure of striated muscle and smooth muscle function: polymyositis. This HRM color contour was recorded from a patient with polymyositis who complained of dysphagia. Resting UES pressure is low, and peristalsis in the striated muscle esophagus is very weak (*arrowhead*). There is no peristalsis in the smooth muscle esophagus.

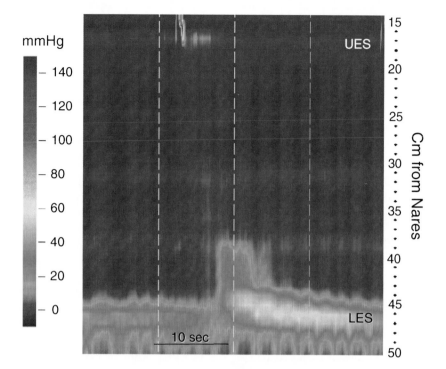

Fig. 2.28. Failure of striated muscle and smooth muscle function: myasthenia gravis. This HRM color contour was recorded from a patient with myasthenia gravis who complained of dysphagia and cough. Resting UES pressure is very low, and peristalsis is absent in the striated and smooth muscle esophagus. Resting LES pressure is normal and the LES relaxation is present.

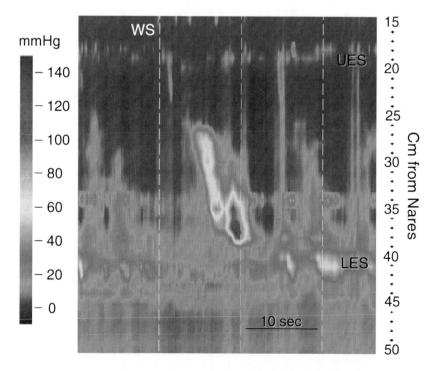

Fig. 2.29. Failure of striated muscle function: radiation injury. This HRM color contour was recorded from a patient with dysphagia and cough who received radiation to the neck as treatment for laryngeal cancer. WS indicates the timing of a wet swallow. Resting UES pressure is very low, and there is essentially no motor activity in the pharynx or striated muscle esophagus. Esophageal and LES motor function are preserved.

by conventional manometry. This is a normal mechanism of reflux in health and when excessive in GERD.

The images shown in Fig. 2.31 are an example of deglutitive inhibition (the double swallow). Propagation of the first primary peristaltic wave was attenuated by a second closely timed dry swallow. Also the second swallow did not generated a peristaltic sequence in the smooth muscle esophagus. This is why it is important to take single wet swallows at 20-30 second intervals during manometric testing. In this situation, the first peristaltic sequence is blocked by the subsequent swallow because of inhibitory mechanisms activated by the second swallow. Since UES motor activity is not continuously monitored, double swallows may not be appreciated and misinterpretation of esophageal function may occur.

High-resolution manometry makes it easy to identify secondary peristalsis (Fig. 2.32). Secondary peristalsis occurs in the absence of a swallow. Typically, secondary peristalsis is a normal mechanism to clear the esophagus of acid, air, or an uncleared bolus from a failed primary peristaltic attempt. Opening of the UES indicates a swallow occured, but no primary peristalsis followed. Almost 15 seconds later, peristaltic sequence occurred, but it was not preceded opening of the UES. This means the second peristalsis was not initiated by a swallow. This is not easily seen with conventional manometry because there is no simultaneous recording from all segments of the esophagus.

Rumination syndrome is a very difficult diagnosis to make since there is no firm diagnostic test. Figure 2.33 shows recordings from a patient with rumination syndrome. The conventional manometry is difficult to interpret. The HRM contour shows the forced regurgitation event, the mechanism of rumination. The marked rise in intraabdominal pressure distinguished rumination from a belch (TLESR)(compare fig. 2.37).

Dysphagia lusoria is a condition that results from vascular compression of the esophagus. Often this is due to the aortic arch but can be due to other anomalous vessels. The difficulty making this diagnosis is that some vascular compression of the esophagus may normally be seen on barium swallow. Ideally, one would like to see hold up of the bolus behind the vessel to accurately make the diagnosis. Vascular pulsations, and pressurization of the esophagus above the lesion suggest the diagnosis (Fig. 2.34). Traditional manometry with sensors that are not closely spaced may miss the diagnosis.

Obesity surgery is very common, and one of the frequently used surgical techniques is the laparoscopic gastric band. Figure 2.35 shows conventional and high-resolution images from a patient with dysphagia after a gastric band. The tracing shows the motor impairments that can result from a tight band.

Traditional manometric techniques can rarely identify an esophageal stricture or distinguish a stricture from a hiatal hernia. The HRM color contour helps make the distinction. Figure 2.36 comes from a patient with a hiatal hernia and distal esophageal stricture. The diaphragm, LES and stricture can be distinguished. The failure of peristalsis and isobaric pressure waves above the stricture look like achalasia. This motor abnormality suggests that the patient has a chronic esophageal obstruction.

Fig. 2.38 to 2.41 are a collection of images that demonstrate miscellaneous findings obtained by HRM, highlighting the diagnostic capability of this technique.

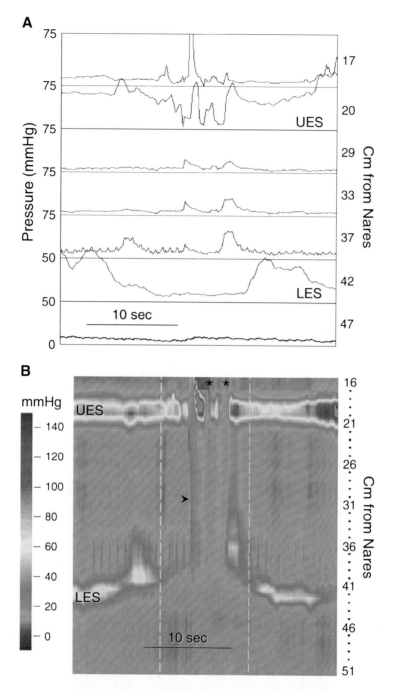

Fig. 2.30. Transient LES relaxation (TLESR) associated with a swallow. (A) This esophageal manometry displayed as a conventional manometry in line mode is difficult to interpret, even when motor activity can be seen simultaneously from the UES to LES. Remember that with conventional manometry techniques we do not record concurrently from the LES, esophagus, and UES. Instead we see the motor activity at the five distal recording sites of this recording. In that circumstance, this motor activity might be misinterpreted as repetitive swallowing, or failed peristalsis with low amplitude, simultaneous, repetitive pressure waves. (B) The HRM color contour gives more insight into the genesis of this motor activity. First, there is shortening of the esophagus that is seen as a proximal migration of the yellow color band that represents resting LES pressure. This is followed by a TLESR. Esophageal shortening often accompanies TLESRs. Next there is a swallow and accompanying intraesophageal (bolus) pressure (*arrowhead*). Following the swallow, the UES opens twice briefly without swallowing (*). Notice that with opening of the UES intraesophageal pressure drops promptly, which is seen as a simultaneous change in color to a darker blue. This indicates venting of the esophagus. Shortly thereafter there is an isolated contraction in the distal smooth muscle esophagus. Finally, the esophagus lengthens and regains its resting tone. This complex motor event is easily understood with HRM.

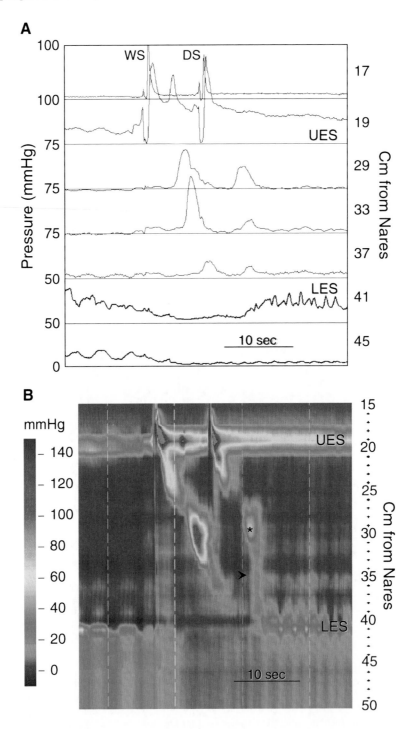

Fig. 2.31. Deglutitive inhibition. (A) A recording displayed in line mode to simulate a conventional manometry. There is a WS followed shortly by a dry swallow (DS). The WS generates a peristaltic sequence that diminishes in amplitude in the distal esophagus. The DS produces a simultaneous pressure event that may be interpreted by some as "simultaneous" contraction. Remember, that with standard manometry techniques simultaneous recordings of UES and smooth muscle esophageal motor function are not obtained. Thus, it may not be apparent that the simultaneous pressure event is produced by a swallow. (B) More details of these motor events are discerned with

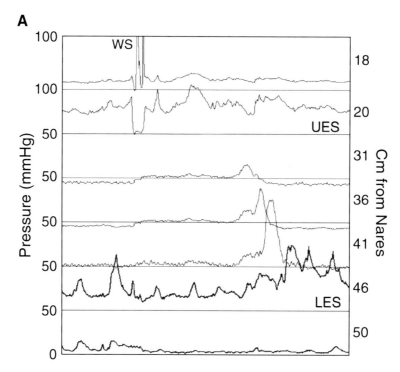

Fig. 2.32. Secondary peristalsis. (A) An esophageal manometry from a patient with dysphagia following Nissen fundoplication displayed in line mode as a conventional manometry tracing. There is peristalsis in the distal esophagus, but it appears to be delayed following the WS. The resting LES pressure is normal, but it is not clear whether LES relaxation is appropriate. (B) The HRM color contour provides more information regarding this motor event. The WS initiates peristalsis in the striated muscle esophagus (*), but no peristaltic activity is generated in the smooth muscle segment. Several seconds later another peristaltic sequence occurs in the striated muscle, but it is not preceded by swallowing. It is, however, followed by normal peristalsis in the smooth muscle esophagus. Esophageal peristalsis not associated with swallowing is called secondary peristalsis. Distending the esophagus produces it. There is an increase in intraesophageal (bolus) pressure (*white arrowhead*) produced by the WS. It is seen as a simultaneous change in color to a lighter blue that coincides temporally with opening of the UES. Notice that the bolus is not cleared; the blue color does not become darker again, until the secondary peristaltic pressure wave passes. The green band of color, which indicates resting LES pressure, does not shift toward the blue hue, which indicates intragastric pressure. This means there is incomplete LES relaxation. Notice that bolus pressure increases near the end of the peristaltic sequence. This is seen as a change from blue to green (*black arrowhead*). The rise in intraesophageal pressure results from compression of the bolus against a closed GE junction, most likely due to obstruction produced by the fundoplication. Incomplete LES relaxation and high bolus pressures are often seen following fundoplication.

Fig. 2.31. (continued) the HRM color contour. What starts out as normal peristalsis with the WS is dramatically attenuated following the DS. This is a phenomenon long known as deglutitive inhibition. It occurs because swallowing initiates a simultaneous wave of inhibition along the smooth muscle esophagus. Thus, the DS attenuates or blocks any ongoing esophageal motor function. The simultaneous pressure event following the DS is produced by an isolated contraction in the proximal smooth muscle esophagus (*) and an associated isobaric pressure wave in the more distal esophagus (*arrowhead*).

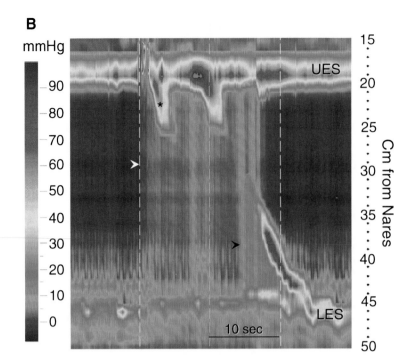

Fig. 2.32. (continued)

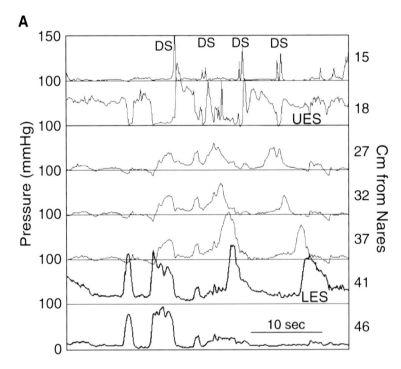

Fig. 2.33. Rumination syndrome. This study was done to evaluate a college student for gastroesophageal reflux. (A) This esophageal manometry displayed as a conventional manometry in line mode is quite complex and confusing, even when motor activity can be seen concurrently from the UES to LES. With conventional manometry techniques we would see only data from the five distal recording sites, making it a daunting manometry for all but the most expert manometrist. (B) The HRM contour plot makes interpreting these motor events much easier. The UES opens spontaneously on two occasions (*). Each UES opening is associated temporally with a sharp rise in intragastric pressure (**). The second rise in intragastric pressure generates a retrograde pressure wave (bolus) moving up the esophagus (*arrowhead*). This pattern is different from the transient LES relaxations in

B

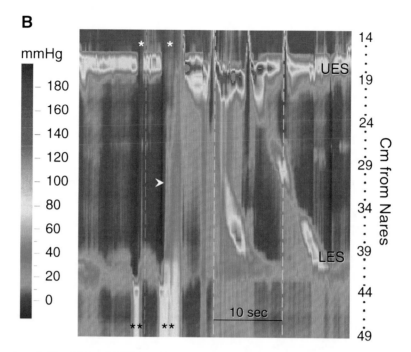

Fig. 2.33. (continued) Figs 2.30 and 2.37, in which retrograde bolus movement is not associated with an increase in intragastric pressure. Regurgitation of gastric contents is followed by several dry swallows that clear the intraesophageal bolus. Bolus clearance is seen as a drop in intraesophageal pressure following a peristaltic sequence.

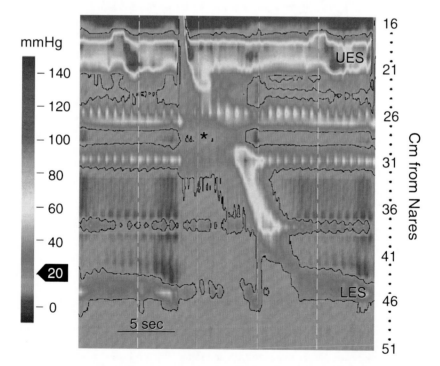

Fig. 2.34. Dysphagia lusoria. This HRM color contour was recorded from a patient with dysphagia and an aberrant right subclavian artery. There are narrow segments of elevated resting intraesophageal pressure located at 26 and 31 cm from the nares. They exhibit synchronous, rhythmic pressure changes at a rate of about 80 per minute. This indicates that they are caused by cardiovascular structures. Black lines bordering the color contours are isobaric pressure lines generated by the computer to indicate when and where the pressure is 20 mmHg. Inside these lines the pressure is >20 mmHg and outside the lines it is <20 mmHg. Notice that the intrabolus pressure is higher cephalad to the pressure zones (*arrowhead*), suggesting a relative obstruction to propulsion of the water bolus.

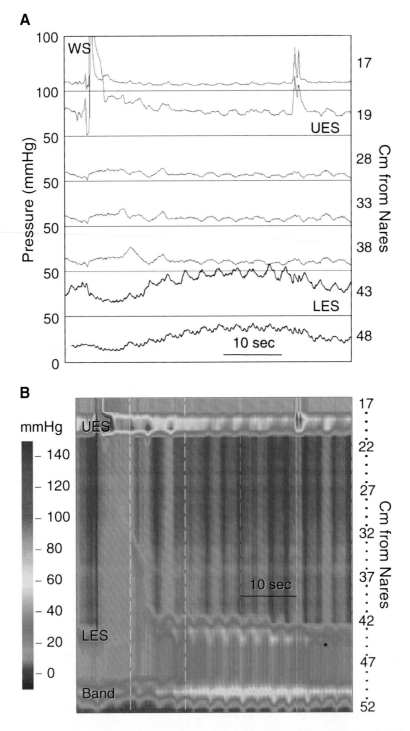

Fig. 2.35. Tight lap band. (A) In this line mode recording we see ineffective or failed peristalsis. The LES is below the diaphragm. Its resting pressure seems to be in the high normal range, and its relaxation approximates an elevated intragastric pressure. Notice that both LES and intragastric pressures are elevated following the WS. (B) In the HRM color contour the same WS. The WS generated an abortive (failed) peristaltic sequence. There are two high-pressure zones located around 43 to 44 cm and 50 to 51 cm from the nares. The upper high-pressure zone coincides with the PIP (*), indicating that the diaphragm and LES are at the same location. Therefore, there is no hiatus hernia. The lower high-pressure zone results from constriction of the stomach by a tight lap band. Notice that the gastric pouch pressurizes following the wet swallow. This suggests that it is not emptying appropriately. Failure of esophageal peristalsis like that seen here is a frequent feature of tight lap bands or other esophageal obstructions. The HRM clearly shows the physiological derangements caused by a tight lap band.

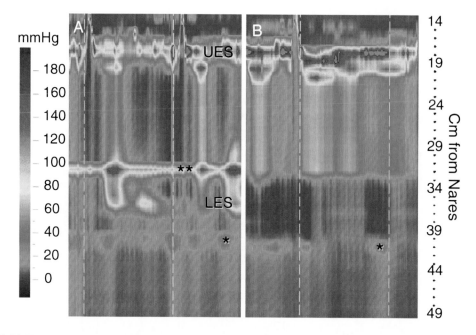

Fig. 2.36. Esophageal stricture. These HRM color contours are from a patient with severe dysphagia and a tight peptic esophageal stricture in the distal esophagus. (A) At the beginning of the study after one WS; (B) at the end of the study. In A, WSs generate simultaneous pressure waves, indicating failure of peristalsis. The LES is located about 36 cm from the nares, and the PIP (*) is at about 40 cm, implying a hiatus hernia. There is another zone of high pressure (**) at about 32 cm from the nares. This high-pressure zone correlates with an endoscopically identified, tight stricture located several centimeters cephalad to the GE junction. At the end of the study, the esophagus is pressurized above the stricture and its motor activity looks like that of achalasia (see Fig. 2.5). There is no peristalsis and there are repetitive, isobaric pressure waves associated with contraction of the striated muscle esophagus.

2.3. Troubleshooting in High-Resolution Manometry of the Esophagus

Technical problems are sometimes encountered during the performance of high-resolution manometry. Some arise from failure of the device, while others occurs with failure of proper catheter placement. The following color contours demonstrate a few examples of such findings. These images will alert readers to the presence of artifacts when performing HRM.

2.3.1. Folded Catheter

Occasionally, when placing a manometry catheter, it will fold on itself. This can happen due to stricture, obstruction, or achalasia. When this happens during conventional manometry, it may be difficult to ascertain what has occurred. In the case of high-resolution color contours, a "butterfly" effect is seen (Fig.2.42). The folded catheter produces a mirror image that looks like a butterfly or Rorschach blot. When this pattern is seen the catheter must be repositioned to avoid damaging it..

2.3.2. Failed Sensor Bank

Sensors in the high-resolution manometry used for the images in this book are closely spaced, and the catheter is assembled from groups of sensors. This

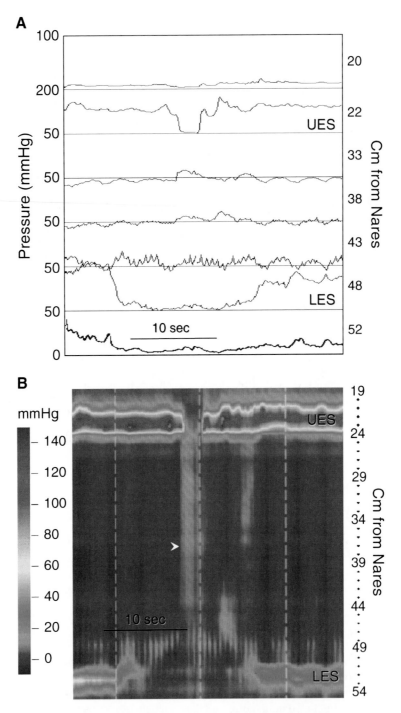

Fig. 2.37. Belch: transient LES relaxation. (A) This manometry displayed in line mode as a conventional manometry reveals a prolonged LES relaxation and UES opening that occurs without associated esophageal or pharyngeal motor activity. These are the motor characteristics of a transient LES relaxation (TLESR). Remember that with conventional manometry techniques we do not record concurrently from the LES, esophagus, and UES. Instead we see the motor activity at the five distal recording sites of this recording. In that circumstance, the motor activity might be misinterpreted as failed peristalsis. The HRM contour reveals the genesis of this motor activity. There are a TLESR, opening of the UES without pharyngeal motor activity, and a transmitted pressure wave in the esophagus that is seen as a simultaneous change in color to a lighter blue (*arrowhead*). This motor complex represents a belch.

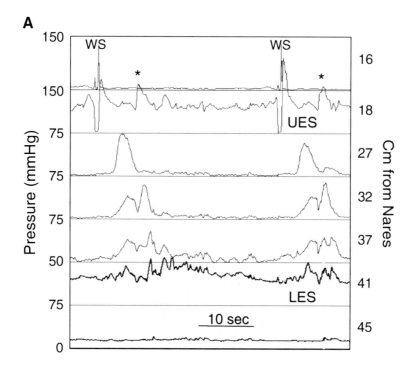

Fig. 2.38. Retrograde bolus movement and incomplete LES relaxation. (A) An esophageal manometry from a patient with dysphagia following Nissen fundoplication displayed in line mode as a conventional manometry tracing. Wet swallows produce what looks like peristalsis in the proximal to middle smooth muscle esophagus that appears to give way to simultaneous repetitive pressure waves in the distal esophagus. The LES does not relax appropriately. Notice that the recording of the UES reveals two pressure waves (*) that are not associated with pharyngeal motor activity, but do correlate temporally with the esophageal pressure wave at 32 cm from the nares. The asterisks were placed to indicate the timing of a gurgling noise coming from the patient's chest. (B) The HRM color contour helps interpret this complex manometry. Wet swallows produce peristalsis in the striated and proximal smooth muscle esophagus. Peristalsis in the proximal smooth muscle segment generates high-amplitude isobaric pressure waves in the more distal esophagus (*arrowheads*). This is seen in the line tracing as the first component of the multipeaked pressure waves recorded in the line mode at 32 and 37 cm from the nares. These isobaric pressures arise from pressurization of the bolus against a closed GE junction. Next the peristalsis breaks down. This is seen as a narrow, vertical band of green between proximal and distal smooth muscle contractions (timing marked by *vertical arrow*). When peristalsis fails the gurgle is heard (*). Notice that the gurgle occurs at the time when there is a simultaneous pressure rise in the proximal esophagus; that is, there is a shift in color from dark to light blue or aqua (*). At the same time pressure in the bolus ahead of the peristaltic pressure wave decreases (*vertical arrow*). These pressure changes indicate that the distal esophagus is being decompressed by bolus escape into the proximal esophagus. Retrograde movement of the bolus produces the gurgle. The two UES pressure peaks seen during the gurgle represent UES contraction at the time pressure went up in the proximal esophagus.

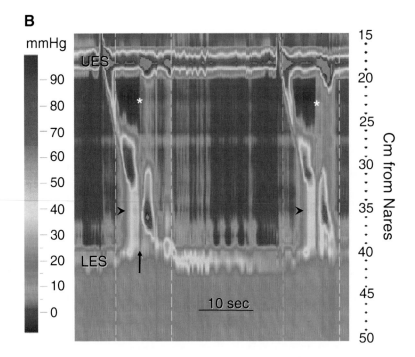

Fig. 2.38. (continued)

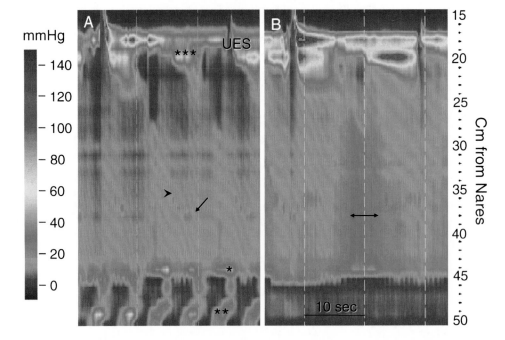

Fig. 2.39. Anastomotic stricture: gastric bypass. These HRM color contours are from a patient with dysphagia, chest pain, and regurgitation after gastric bypass. (A) At the beginning of the study after one WS; (B) at the end of the study. (A) A WS produces weak (ineffective) peristalsis in the smooth muscle esophagus arrowhead). Secondary peristalsis also starts in the striated muscle esophagus (***) without EUS opening, and propagates as ineffective peristalsis in the smooth muscle esophagus. The *arrow* indicates the location of the GE junction. The PIP is not coincident with the GE junction, but cannot be clearly identified. This suggests a hiatus hernia. At 45 cm from the nares, there is a transition above which the intraluminal pressure is higher than below (*). Normally resting intraesophageal pressure is lower than intragastric pressure because intrathoracic pressure is lower than

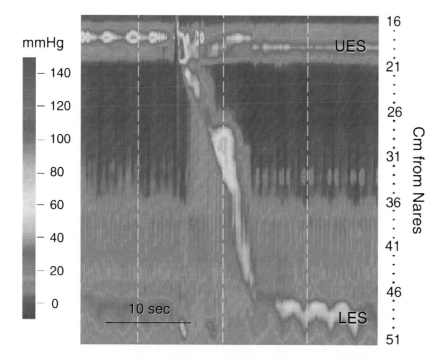

Fig. 2.40. Cardiac compression of the esophagus. This HRM color contour was recorded from a patient with dysphagia and congestive heart failure. There is normal motor function of the UES, LES, and esophagus. Between approximately 36 and 45 cm from the nares there is a zone of elevated resting intraesophageal pressure that changes rhythmically at the heart rate, indicating that it is cardiac in origin.

means that single sensors or a group may fail. Consequently, a single channel, or a series of adjacent channels may not function. Figure 2.43 shows a variety of artifacts produced by sensor failure. These patterns indicate the catheter needs repair or replacement.

2.3.3. Air in the Sheath

Fig. 2.44 demonstrates a peristaltic sequence with air in the hygienic sheath that covers the catheter. This picture is seen when air trapped between the catheter and sheath forced distally by peristalsis to pressurize the sheath.

Fig. 2.39. (continued) intraabdominal pressure (see Fig. 2.2). Higher resting intraesophageal pressures suggest functional (achalasia) or mechanical (stricture, see Fig. 2.37) obstruction. Below the partition, there is a cyclical contractile activity that recurs at about 12 per minute (**). This type of contractile activity is seen in the small bowel during phase III of the migrating myoelectrical complex. At the end of the study, resting intraesophageal pressure and intrabolus pressure produced by peristalsis (*double-headed arrow*) are greater than earlier. These findings suggest obstruction. Notice that the cyclical activity at the bottom of the tracing is gone, indicating passage of the phase III. Endoscopy confirmed a hiatus hernia of the gastric pouch and a stricture at the gastrojejunostomy anastomosis.

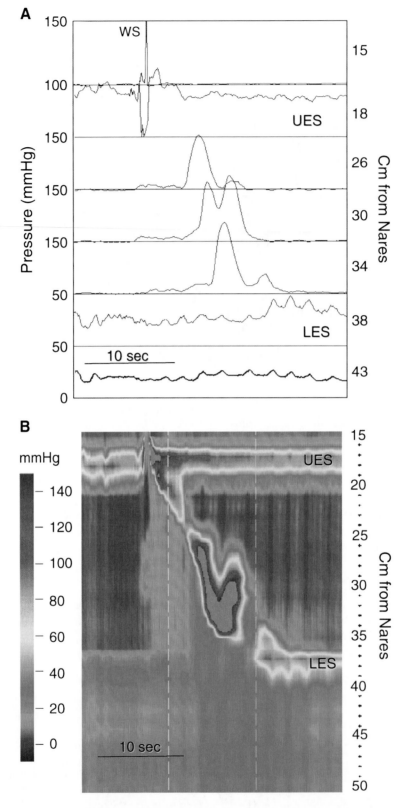

Fig. 2.41. Retrograde peristalsis. (A) The manometry displayed in line mode as a conventional manometry reveals what is commonly referred to as a double-peaked pressure wave at the recording site 30 cm from the nares. The conventional wisdom is that this is a variation of normal esophageal motor function. (B) The HRM color contour reveals that the double-peaked pressure wave is actually retrograde contraction. This is not readily apparent on the conventional tracing because the sensors are to widely spaced to pick it up.

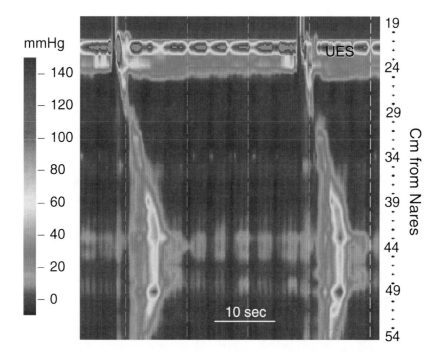

Fig. 2.42. Artifact produced by folded catheter. This HRM contour displays artifact typical of the manometry catheter folded back upon itself. Motor function is normal in the UES and striated muscle esophagus. There is no LES and no PIP. Peristalsis appears normal to about 43 cm from the nares. The pressure is simultaneous from 43 to 49 cm, and below 49 cm there appears to be reverse peristalsis. The color contour from 46 to 54 cm is a mirror image of that from 38 to 46 cm. It looks like a butterfly or Rorschach blot. This is the color contour produced when the catheter is folded upon itself. If this pattern is seen, the catheter should be immediately repositioned to avoid its damage.

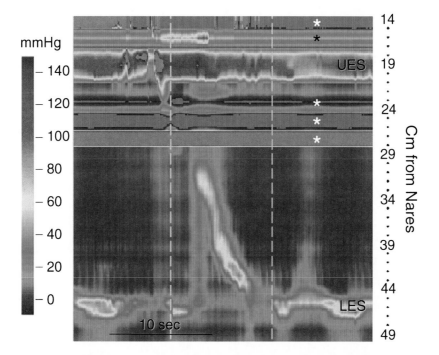

Fig. 2.43. Artifact-produced sensor failure. This HRM contour displays typical artifacts caused by sensor failure (*asterisks*). Sensor failure may be seen as solid bands of color or an irregular "chatter" in the color contour (top of the contour).

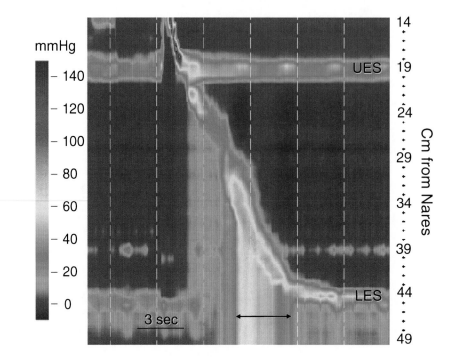

Fig. 2.44. Artifact-produced air entrapment. This HRM contour displays a typical artifact caused by air being trapped in a protective sheath over the catheter. As peristalsis in the smooth muscle esophagus progresses, a very high bolus pressure develops and is transmitted all the way to the end of the catheter (*double-headed arrow*). This is the type of artifact seen when there is air between the protective sheath and catheter. It is produced by a peristaltic contraction squeezing the entrapped air toward the distal pressure sensors.

Gastric/Small Bowel Manometry

Manometry of the antrum and small bowel has been performed for several decades with the same technologies used for esophageal manometry. However, the patterns of contractions in these segments are more complex than those of the esophagus, and the advantages of high-resolution manometry (HRM) over other recording techniques are best highlighted in this segment of the gastrointestinal (GI) tract. Antroduodenal manometry is performed over a number of hours during fasting, to capture components of the migrating motor complex (MMC), and following a meal. Contraction sequences are antegrade or retrograde, propagate over various lengths of bowel, and occur irregularly, producing numerous pressure events. Conventional manometry uses a limited number of widely spaced sensors. The large amounts of water perfused through catheter side holes during a study may affect intestinal motility. Widely spaced side holes make it difficult to assess patterns of propagation of individual or groups of contractions. Consequently, evaluation of antroduodenal manometry is primarily qualitative, relying on visual recognition of characteristic contractile patterns that occur during fasting and postprandial. Some quantitative analysis, such as a motility index, can be made.

High-resolution manometry offers a significant advantage in assessing contractile events in the small bowel and stomach. The greatest advantage is the ability to observe and analyze individual or groups of contractile sequences, and their direction and length of spread, regardless of how "busy" the tracing is. Better assessment of contractile sequences can offer a better understanding of flow that ultimately results from such sequences. This chapter demonstrates manometry of the stomach and duodenum. Figure 3.1 is a radiographic image of the HRM catheter in position for antroduodenal manometry test.

3.1. Normal Gastric and Small Bowel High-Resolution Manometry

The stomach and small bowel are integrated functionally to facilitate digestion. This integration includes feedback mechanisms that modulate gastric activity at any given moment, depending on the amount of caloric material entering the small bowel. The distal stomach and the small bowel generate stereo-typic patterns of motor activity that serve as an index of the integrity of their neuromuscular apparatus. These patterns, observed in the fasting and

J. Conklin, *Color Atlas of High Resolution Manometry*,
DOI: 10.1007/978-0-387-88295-6_3, © Springer Science+Business Media, LLC 2009

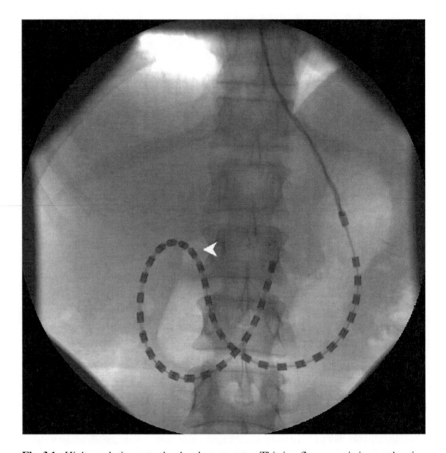

Fig. 3.1. High-resolution antroduodenal manometry. This is a fluoroscopic image showing placement of the high-resolution manometry catheter for antroduodenal manometry. The dark rectangles are individual pressure sensors. The recording segment of the catheter is composed of 36 closely spaced, circumferential, pressure sensors spaced at a distance of 1 cm from center to center, providing a sensing length of 35 cm. It spans from the stomach to the level of the ligament of Treitz. Because a number of closely spaced sensors straddle the pylorus, appreciation of this transition zone (*arrowhead*) does not require special devices (such as a sleeve). Similarly, movement of the catheter does not affect recording from the antrum, which can happen, for example, after a meal.

fed states, have distinct features and properties that are vital to normal gut function.

3.1.1. Fasting State

The fasting period is characterized by the migrating myoelectrical complex (MMC). It is a cyclical event that consists of three phases. The most distinct is termed phase III, a band of regular phasic pressure events that can initiate in the stomach or in the small bowel, but the highest prevalence is at the ligament of Treitz. Gastric contractions occur at a rate of three per minute, while the rate in the proximal small bowel is about 12 per minute. This distinct motor event is highly propulsive, and is considered to be the "housekeeper," cleansing the stomach and the small bowel of all food material that is left behind after digestion and absorption are completed. Figure 3.2 shows a typical phase III involving the antrum and duodenum. This phase is easily recognized by traditional manometry (Fig. 3.2A), but the HRM tracing provides information about the spread of individual contractions that is not readily apparent with conventional manometry (Fig. 3.2B).

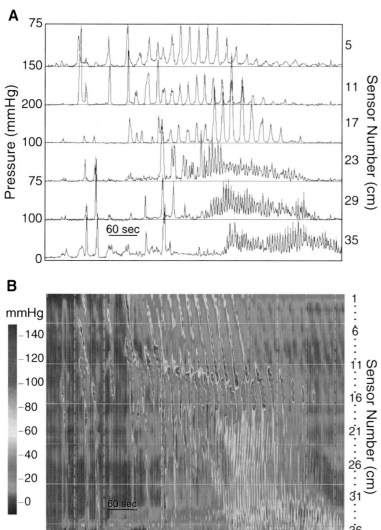

Fig. 3.2. Phase III of the migrating motor complex (MMC) in the antrum and duodenum. (A) An antroduodenal manometry displayed in line mode was recorded from the catheter positioned in Fig. 3.1. It demonstrates a phase III of the MMC. Pressures are displayed from sensors spaced at 5-cm intervals to approximate the look of a conventional antroduodenal manometry. The top three channels display antral motor activity: high-amplitude peristaltic contractions at three cycles per min (cpm). The bottom three channels display duodenal motor activity: peristaltic contractions at 12 cpm. It is relatively easy to appreciate the direction the phase III complex and gastric pressure waves propagate, but very difficult to evaluate propagation of duodenal pressure waves. (B) The high-resolution manometry (HRM) color contour of the same data. The location of the pylorus, as estimated from the fluoroscopic image, is in the neighborhood of sensors 16 and 17. The HRM contour provides a more detailed depiction of antroduodenal motor function. The propagation of individual contractions can be discerned, even in this condensed tracing.

Figure 3.3 expands the time base of Fig. 3.2 to further highlight the ability of HRM to provide clear information on pyloric function and antroduodenal coordination. The role of the pylorus in gastric emptying and gastroduodenal motor function is not fully understood, in part because of technical difficulties. The gastroduodenal junction is difficult to study with traditional manometry. Thus, specifically designed catheters incorporating sleeve devices were used for this purpose. However, gastric contraction or relaxation, particularly following a meal, can displace the catheter, so that it loses contact with the pylorus. This problem is circumvented by the HRM catheter. The high-resolution technique provides simultaneous views of the stomach, pylorus, and duodenum as demonstrated in Fig. 3.3B. Figure 3.4 shows a variation in the spread of contractions in phase III that cannot be appreciated with traditional manometry.

A period of quiescence following phase III, called phase I, may or may not be present during the daytime. During phase I, less than three phasic pressure events are expected to occur per 10-minute interval. The intermittent motor activity observed between phases I and III is defined as phase II, and it makes up most of the duration of the MMC cycle in the fasting state. Contractions in phase II can propagate antegrade or retrograde over various distances. Those that propagate aborally over long distance are highly propulsive. Figure 3.5 shows cotractions that in frequency, the details of propagation are difficult to discern in the traditional manometry (Fig. 3.6).

3.1.2. Fed State

In the fed state, motor activity serves to optimize the digestive processes by grinding, sieving, and mixing gastrointestinal contents. Contractile activity is increased in both the stomach and duodenum. Antral contractions serve mainly to grind and triturate ingested food to particles that are small enough to traverse the pyloric region. In contrast, contractile activity in the small bowel is primarily suited for mixing of bowel contents, providing adequate contact with the absorbing surface of the bowel. Figure 3.7 depicts motor activity following a meal. The HRM tracing clearly shows the stationary and bidirectional contractions observed after a meal.

In the reminder of this chapter we show intermediate and abnormal patterns of contractions. Figure 3.8 is an example of *cluster activity* observed in phase II of the MMC. This term refers to groups of contractions, of short duration, separated by quiescence. This activity can be seen in healthy subjects, and in conditions such as the irritable bowel syndrome. Figure 3.9 demonstrates fasting antral activity in a patient with short bowel syndrome. There is continuous contractile activity, unrelated to phase III of the MMC. This phenomenon is likely related to a loss of intestinal inhibition of gastric motor activity. Figure 3.10 shows a retrograde propagation of phase III in a patient after gastric bypass operation for obesity. The patient developed symptoms of nausea and vomiting immediately after the operation. Standard imaging studies did not reveal the problem. Following revision of the Roux limb, symptoms completely resolved.

Much is still unknown about the complex contractile events in the stomach and small bowel, primarily due to limitations of existing manometric techniques. Thus far, there is very little experience with HRM technology in GI motor disorders. The advantages of HRM technology over traditional mano-metry (Table 3.1), and in particular the ability to observe individual

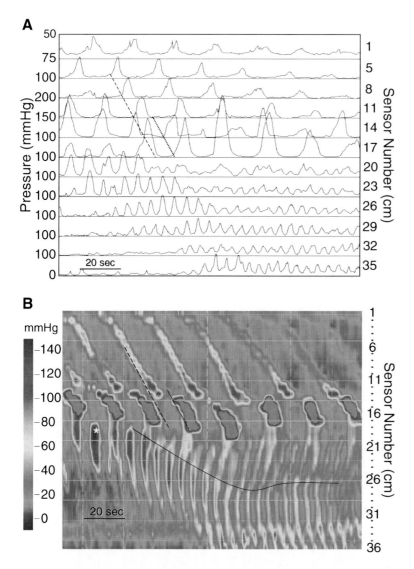

Fig. 3.3. Phase III of the migrating motor complex (MMC). (A) A more detailed line mode plot of the data in Fig. 3.2. The time base is expanded threefold, and sensor spacing is decreased to 3 cm, except between sensors 1 and 5. Gastric motor activity is depicted in the top six channels and duodenal motor activity in the bottom 6. The *dashed line* was placed to identify the takeoff point of peristaltic pressure waves in the stomach. It is easy to follow propagation from channels 5 to 11. The peristaltic waves recorded at sensors 14 and 17 appear out of phase with those above them, because their takeoff points (*dotted line*) are offset from the *dashed line*. It remains difficult to determine the direction of propagation in the duodenum. (B) The HRM color contour from the same data gives an unambiguous picture of phase III motor activity. The *dashed* and *dotted lines* correlate spatially and temporally with those in the line-mode plot (A). The HRM contour identifies propagated gastric pressure waves (*dashed line*). They appear to slow or cease just prior to a vigorous contraction that occurs in the most distal 3 to 5 cm of the antropyloric region (*dotted line*). The color contour demonstrates how the pressure wave identified in channels 14 and 17 of the line plot are associated with the preceding pressure wave in channels 5, 8, and 11. The direction of duodenal peristalsis during phase III is easily discerned with the HRM contour (B). Duodenal peristalsis (*) propagates antegrade at the beginning of this phase III. As time progresses, retrograde peristalsis appears, and the point from which it is initiated moves retrograde (*solid line*). This means that the position of dominant pacemaker activity is changing over time. Also, notice that the velocity of peristalsis varies along the duodenal segment.

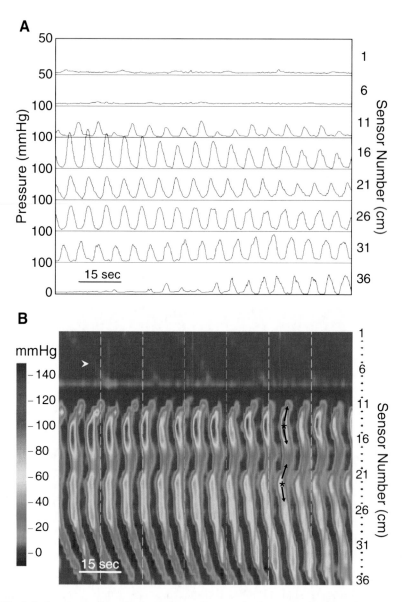

Fig. 3.4. Duodenal phase III in a healthy subject. (A) This antroduodenal manometry is displayed in line mode to simulate a traditional tracing of phase III in the duodenum. The propagation pattern of contractile sequences is difficult to reliably determine. (B) The HRM color contour of the same tracing makes it easy to discern the complex pattern of propagation. Very low amplitude pressure waves are seen in the stomach (*arrowhead*). There are two pacemaker foci in the duodenum (*) from which pressure waves propagate antegrade and retrograde (*arrows*). Also notice that individual duodenal pressure waves propagate at varying velocities over different duodenal segments.

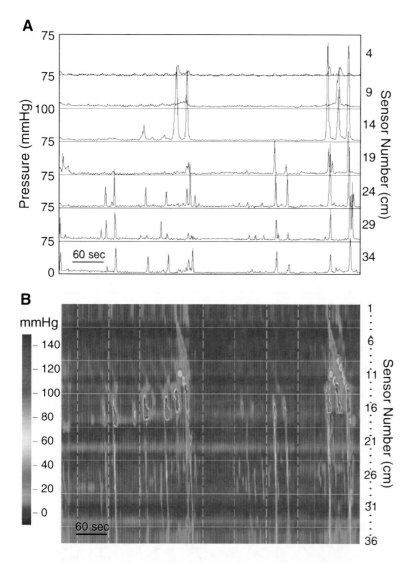

Fig. 3.5. Phase II of the MMC in a healthy subject. (A) This antroduodenal manometry is displayed in line mode to simulate a traditional tracing of phase II of the MMC. The top three channels are from the stomach and the bottom four from the duodenum. There are a number of long duodenal contractile sequences propagating antegrade. Some are associated with an antral component. Because individual sequences are separated by periods of quiescence, they can easily be observed in the traditional tracing.

contractile sequences with great clarity, suggest that this technology can greatly advance our understanding of gut motor physiology. It is hoped that it will also provide better understanding of disease states, and the ability to better distinguish health from disease.

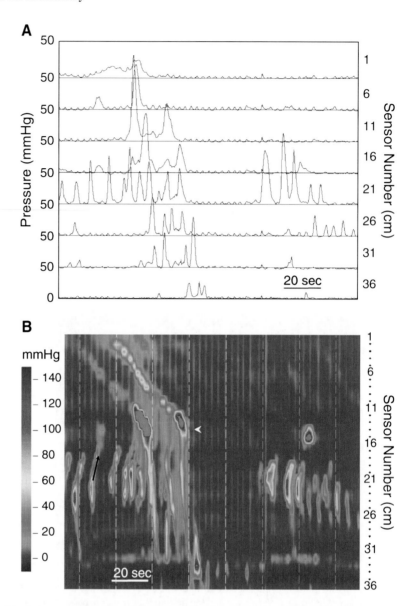

Fig. 3.6. Phase II of the MMC in a healthy subject. (A) This antroduodenal manometry is displayed in line mode to simulate a traditional tracing of phase II of the MMC. The top four channels are from the stomach and the bottom 4 from the duodenum. With more duodenal activity it becomes difficult to determine the direction in which duodenal pressure waves spread. (B) The HRM color contour of the same tracing makes it easier to discern the complex pattern of propagation. Antropyloric peristaltic sequences are followed by duodenal contractions that propagate over long lengths (*arrowhead*). Again, notice that retrograde propagation is common in the proximal duodenum.

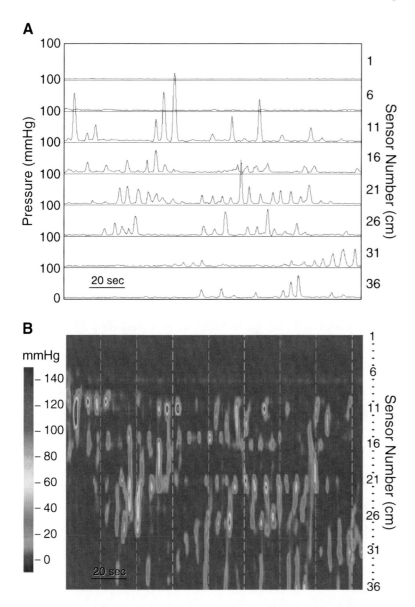

Fig. 3.7. Motor function after a meal. (A) This antroduodenal manometry is displayed in line mode to simulate a traditional tracing of the fed pattern. It was obtained more than an hour after a light meal. The top two channels are from the stomach and the bottom six from the duodenum. The directional spread of contractile sequences is particularly difficult to determine in the postprandial period with its typical "busy" contractile activity, when viewing displays of traditional recording. This is true even when the tracing is greatly expanded, as it is here. (B) The HRM color contour allows a detailed analysis of each and every sequence. Contractions are increased in number. Most are stationary, and occupy short intestinal segments. Propagated contractions spread antegrade and retrograde. A number of stationary contractions occur simultaneously along the duodenum. This pattern is likely to result in bidirectional flow of intestinal contents over short distances, resulting primarily in mixing of digesta.

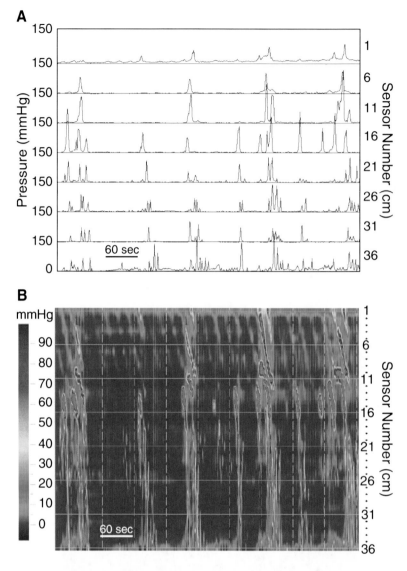

Fig. 3.8. Cluster activity in a healthy subject. (A) This antroduodenal manometry is displayed in line mode to simulate a traditional tracing of phase II of the MMC. The top three channels are from the stomach and the bottom four from the duodenum. Groups of duodenal contractions of short duration occur at the maximal frequency of the duodenum and propagated over various lengths of intestine. They are separated by short periods of quiescence. This activity can be seen in health, usually during phase II of the MMC when subjects are awake, and also in conditions such as the irritable bowel syndrome. (B) The color contour in the HRM display clearly shows propagation of clusters as well as individual pressure contractions.

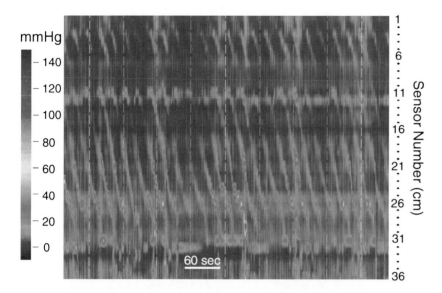

Fig. 3.9. Antral motor activity during fasting in a patient with short bowel syndrome. The HRM display demonstrates continuous gastric propagated contractions at a frequency ofv about 3 cpm. This is distinctly abnormal when contrasted with the usual intermittent activity during fasting. This likely represents a loss of intestinal inhibitory mechanisms that modulate gastric motility resulting from removal of the distal half of the small bowel.

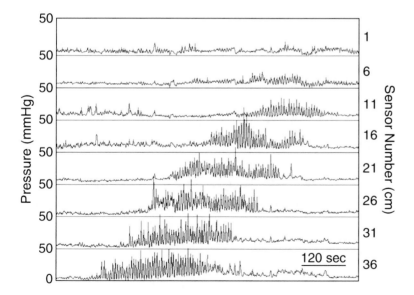

Fig. 3.10. Phase III of the migrating motor complex in a patient post–Roux-en-Y gastric bypass. Recording is obtained from the jejunum (Roux limb). (A,B) Both displays show a phase III with a retrograde propagation. The reason for this striking phenomenon was that the Roux limb was anastomosed in a reverse fashion. Symptoms of nausea and vomiting resolved immediately after revision of the Roux limb.

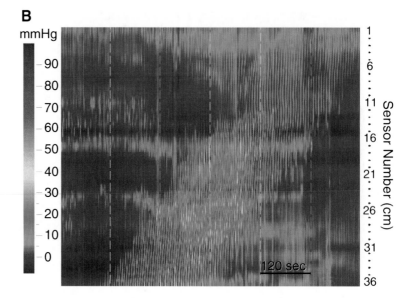

Fig. 3.10. (continued)

Table 3.1. Pros and cons of conventional versus high-resolution manometry of the stomach and small bowel.

Conventional manometry	High-resolution manometry
Wide spacing of channels (10–15 cm apart)	Tight spacing (1.0 cm apart)
Can only evaluate long segment antegrade and retrograde contractions due to wide spacing	Can see short and long segment antegrade and retrograde contractions
See wave forms but often uncertain of direction of contractions (retrograde vs. antegrade)	Can more clearly discern direction of contractions
Pyloric pressures not easy to locate	Pylorus readily apparent
Easier to place fluoroscopically due to stiffness of catheter and channel for wire	More difficult to place due to softer tube structure

Anorectal Manometry

4.1. Normal High-Resolution Anorectal Manometry

Anorectal manometry requires a different design of catheter, depicted in Fig. 4.1. A set of 10 closely spaced sensors spans a length of 6 cm. It simultaneously captures pressure data from the rectum, anal and atmospere. A second array of sensors, located close to the tip, captures intrarectal pressure. A balloon attached to metal rings (arrow) serves to elicit the rectoanal inhibitory reflex, and also is used for assessment of rectal sensation.

4.1.1. Normal Anal Sphincter

Throughout this book, displays of conventional manometry are contrasted with those of high-resolution manometry, to allow comparison and illustrate differences between techniques. The same approach is used in examining anorectal manometry. High-resolution manometry provides a clear display of pressure events in the anal canal and in the rectum that is unaffected by catheter displacement resulting from movement of the pelvic floor. However, in the anorectum, the advantage of HRM over traditional manometry may not be as pronounced as in the esophagus and antroduodenum. This is due to the short length of the anal canal, allowing for the placement of a few closely spaced sensors in catheters built for traditional manometry. Also, anorectal manometry captures primarily sphincteric motor events, which have a limited variety. Anorectal manometry with the HRM catheter is conducted in a manner similar to that of traditional manometry. Once a baseline anal pressure is obtained, a number of tests are conducted to assess sphincter strength, defecation dynamics, and reflex mechanisms.

Baseline resting pressure depends primarily on the resting tone of the internal anal sphincter and is measured first (Fig. 4.2). This is then followed by the voluntary squeeze effort by the patient, to tighten the anal sphincter (external sphincter). Figure 4.3A depicts a typical record of a normal anal squeeze in conventional manometry. In HRM, color changes indicates variations in pressure (Fig. 4.3B).

The second phase of the procedure is the defecatory maneuver, a test of simulated defecation. During this maneuver, the high-resolution catheter allows visualization of anal canal and intrarectal pressures simultaneously. Normally,

J. Conklin, *Color Atlas of High Resolution Manometry*,
DOI: 10.1007/978-0-387-88295-6_4, © Springer Science + Business Media, LLC 2009

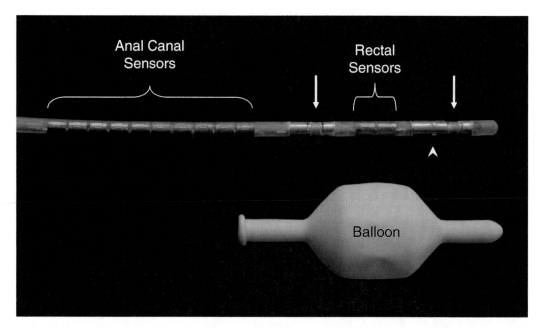

Fig. 4.1. High-resolution anorectal manometry catheter. The high-resolution manometry catheter pictured here is 4.2 mm in diameter and consists of 12 circumferential, solid-state, pressure sensors (copper colored bands). Ten of the sensors comprising the anal-sensing segment are spaced at 6-mm intervals from center to center (anal sensors). This gives the catheter a recording segment of 5.6 cm. There are 3 cm between this anal sensing segment and a pair of sensors located in a balloon during the study (rectal sensors). These sensors measure pressure in the rectum and in the inflated balloon. Metal rings are used to tie the balloon onto the catheter (*arrows*), and there are also air insufflation ports (*arrowhead*). Each individual sensor detects pressure from 12 loci around its circumference. Computer processing of signals coming from pressure sensing elements allows average circumferential pressures over recording segments to be displayed in real time and recorded for subsequent analysis.

the anal sphincter relaxes, while intrarectal pressure increases, mimicking the pressure events that occur during evacuation of stool. Figures 4.4 and 4.5 are examples of this maneuver. Artifacts caused by movement of sphicteric structures relative to the catheter can occur during anorectal manometry, as they due during esophageal manometry (see Fig. 2.5B in Chapter 2). Figure 4.6 is an example of such movement during attempted defecation that may wrongly be interpreted as showing adequate relaxation of the sphincter.

The study is usually concluded with graded rectal balloon distention. This maneuver serves two purposes: assessment rectal sensation and elicitation of the rectoanal inhibitory reflex (RAIR). Typically, volumes of air that induce a constant sensation of pressure and urge to deficate are determined. Reduced rectal sensation can be corrected by biofeedback, a therapy that can be helpful in both constipation and incontinence. Internal anal sphincter relaxation in response to balloon inflation, the RAIR, (Figs. 4.7 and 4.8) tests the integrety of the myentreic plexus. The relaxation increases as a function of balloon volume (Fig. 4.7). Anal pressure is reduced, but not abolished because the external sphincter continues to maintain its tone. This is easily seen in figure 4.7. Loss of the RAIR is seen Hirschprung's disease or megarectum

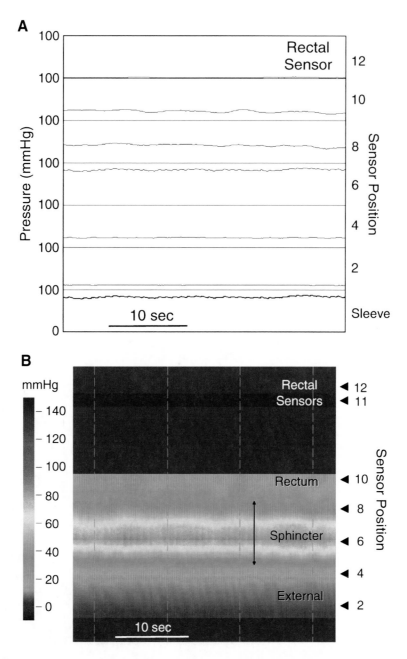

Fig. 4.2. Resting anorectal motor function. Conventional anorectal manometry systems record and display intraluminal pressures from unidirectional or circumferential sensors spaced at 1- to 2-cm intervals. (A) This recording was made with a high-resolution anorectal manometry catheter and recording system (Manoscan™, Sierra Scientific Instruments), but it is displayed in the line mode. Five of 10 anal canal recording channels and one intrarectal (balloon) channel were chosen for display to mimic what is seen with conventional manometry systems. Pressure is on the y-axis, time is on the x-axis, and pressure tracings are stacked vertically. The numbers to the right of the graphic indicate sensor position. The spacing between displayed sensors is 12 mm. Sensor 2 is the most external and sensor 10 is the most internal of the anal sensing array. The tracing labeled rectal sensor (position 12) is a sensor in a balloon about 3.6 cm cephalad to the anal sensing segment. The bottom trace is from an electronic (virtual) sleeve that measures pressure simultaneously across the entire anal canal and displays the highest pressure in the anal canal at each time point. (B) The high-resolution color contour of the same recording. Pressure is represented by color, with the color bar to the left indicating the relationship between color and pressure. Sensor location is on the y-axis and time is on the x-axis. Sensors 1 to 10 are spaced at 6-mm intervals, and sensors 11 and 12 are in the balloon 3 cm cephalad to sensor 10. Pressure generated by the resting anal sphincters is seen as a broad band of bright color (*double-headed arrow*).

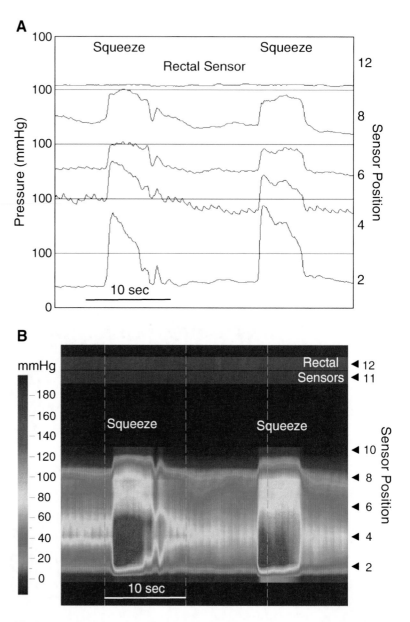

Fig. 4.3. Squeeze maneuver. (A) This anorectal manometry displayed in line mode as a conventional manometry reveals a typical recording obtained from a subject asked to contract the external anal sphincter as if trying to stop the defecation process. The timing of the squeeze is indicated at the top of the tracing (squeeze). Sensors 2 to 8 are in the anal canal, and the pressure they detect increases when the subject is asked to squeeze. (B) The same data are presented as a high-resolution manometry (HRM) color contour. Contraction of the external sphincter and puborectalis is seen as shift to warmer colors. Notice that there is no change in rectal pressure, indicating that there was no Valsalva during the squeeze maneuver.

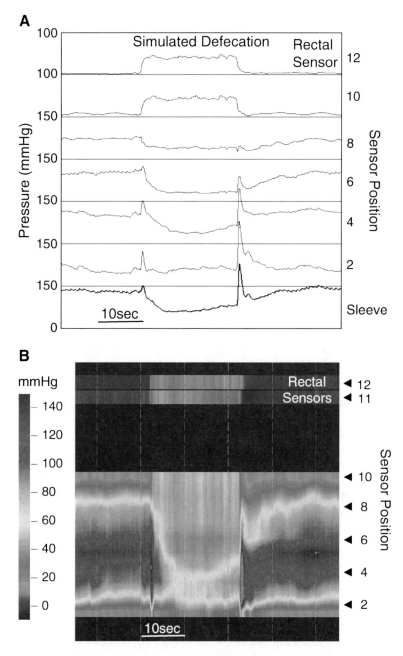

Fig. 4.4. Simulated defecation: the bear-down maneuver. (A) This anorectal manometry displayed in line mode as a conventional manometry demonstrates the response when the subject was asked to bear down as if having a bowel movement. The timing of the maneuver is indicated at the top of the tracing, as simulated defecation. The precise timing is indicated by the rise in intrarectal pressure (channels 10 and 12) produced by the Valsalva maneuver. Relaxation is seen in channels 4 to 8. Notice that relaxation is also seen in the virtual sleeve. This indicates that there was a drop in pressure across the entire anal canal during simulated defecation. (B) The same data are presented as an HRM color contour. The rise in intrarectal pressure produced by the Valsalva maneuver is seen in channels 11 and 12 as a change in color from blue to green. It is also observed with the most internal sensors of the anal canal array (9 and 10). Relaxation of the anal canal musculature is seen as a drop in pressure indicated by color change from violets and reds to yellows and greens.

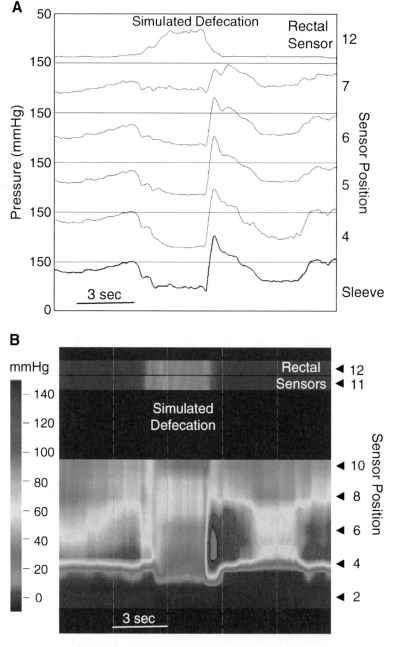

Fig. 4.5. Simulated defecation: the bear-down maneuver. (A) This anorectal manometry displayed in line mode as a conventional manometry is another demonstration of the response when a subject was asked to bear down as if having a bowel movement. This tracing is very similar to that in Fig. 4.4A. Again, relaxation is seen in the virtual sleeve, indicating a drop in pressure across the entire anal canal during simulated defecation. (B) The same data are presented as an HRM color contour. The rise in intrarectal pressure produced by the Valsalva maneuver (channels 11 and 12) is not great, suggesting a poor effort on the part of the subject. Relaxation of the anal canal musculature is seen as a drop in pressure indicated by color change from reds and yellows to yellows and greens.

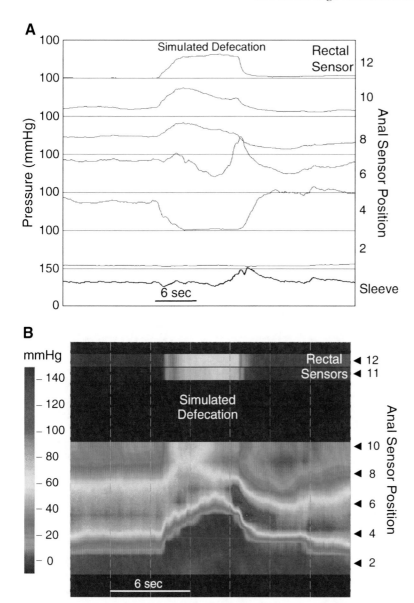

Fig. 4.6. Simulated defecation: catheter movement. (A) This anorectal manometry displayed in line mode as a conventional manometry is another demonstration of the response when a subject was asked to bear down as if having a bowel movement. At first glance it looks as though the anal sphincter relaxes because there is a drop in pressure at channels 4 and 6. Sensor 2 appears to be outside the anal canal, and the identical waveforms in channels 8 and 10 suggest that they are detecting intrarectal pressure. Notice that the virtual sleeve does not register a drop in pressure across the anal canal during simulated defecation. (B) The same data presented as an HRM color contour clarify what is really happening. The HRM contour looks like an arch during simulated defecation, with the color changing from red and yellow to blue at channel 4. This blue represents the pressure outside the anal canal. The color in the arch does not change, indicating that the sphincter is not relaxing. Thus, this HRM contour demonstrates an artifact caused by the catheter being pushed out of the anal canal during simulated defecation. In the conventional line mode, this artifact might well have been interpreted as relaxation.

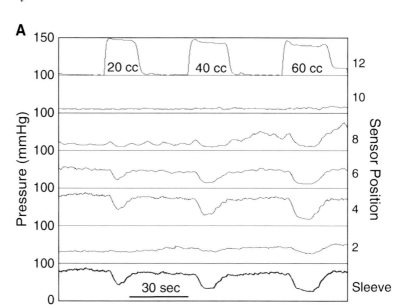

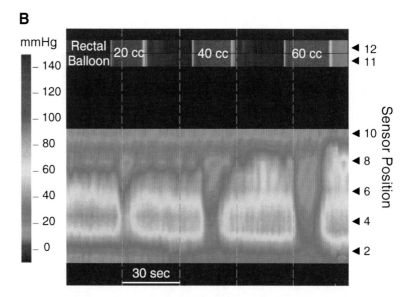

Fig. 4.7. Rectoanal inhibitory reflex. (A) This anorectal manometry displayed in line mode as a conventional manometry demonstrates a normal rectoanal inhibitory reflex (RAIR). To elicit the reflex, air is injected through the catheter into a balloon enclosing the rectal sensors (channels 11 and 12). Balloon distension increases pressure registered by the intrarectal sensors. The volume of air injected is displayed along with the pressure change it induced (sensor 12). Balloon distension normally produces a graded relaxation of the anal canal musculature (channels 4, 6, and 8). (B) The HRM color contour of the same data. It confirms the impression from the line-mode tracing. Relaxation is seen as a change in color from red and yellow to green and blue. Most of the time, the RAIR appears to start on the rectal side of the anal canal and spread caudal as a function of balloon volume. This reflex is mediated at the level of the myenteric plexus and it is the internal anal (smooth muscle) sphincter that relaxes.

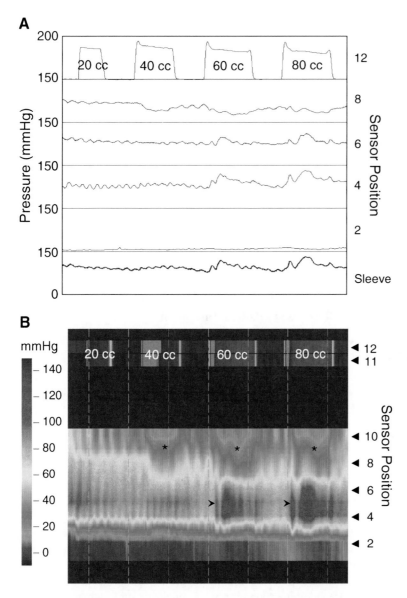

Fig. 4.8. Rectoanal inhibitory and contractile reflexes. (A) This high-resolution anorectal manometry displayed in line mode demonstrates a somewhat atypical response to balloon distension. At first glance it looks as though there is failure of the RAIR. Careful examination demonstrates relaxation in channel 8. (B) The HRM color contour of the same data gives a clear picture of these motor events. The sphincteric segment is quite long, spanning from channel 3 to above channel 10, making it >4.2 cm in length. The RAIR occurs on the rectal side of the anal canal (*), but not across the entire anal canal. Instead, there is an increase in anal canal pressure (*arrowhead*) from contraction of the external anal sphincter. This is the rectoanal contractile reflex. It occurs without the patient sensing rectal fullness or the urge to defecate. Here the response is more vigorous than is usually seen.

4.1.2. Cough Reflex

Another maneuver that is conducted during manometry in some centers is the cough reflex (Fig. 4.9). A sudden rise in intraabdominal pressure, such as occurs during cough, results in an increase in anal pressure caused by contraction of the external sphincter. This is a multi-synaptic sacral reflex that helps to maintain continence, and a useful maneuver when investigating fecal incontinence.

4.1.3. Oscillating Pressure Waves

Figure 4.10 shows ultraslow waves, at a rate of about one per minute. Ultraslow waves occur at a rate of one to two per minute, are usually generate a high basal pressure.

4.1.4. Anoanal Reflex

Figure 4.11 shows the reflex contraction of the external sphincter to slight movement of the catheter. This is easily recognized when performing HRM.

4.1.5. Rectal Response to Balloon Distention

Figures 4.8 and 4.12 demonstrate and contractile response sometimes seen during rectal balloon distention.

4.2. Abnormal High-Resolution Anorectal Manometry

The following subsections discuss a number of disease states that can be recognized during conventional manometry.

4.2.1. Dyssynergic Defecation

This phenomenon, also called anismus, pelvic floor dysfunction, pelvic dyssynergia, and obstructed defecation, is an abnormal response of the anal sphincter during attempted defecation. A number of variations are observed. The typical presentation is shown in Fig. 4.13 and is referred to as type I dyssynergic defecation. It consists of a paradoxical increase in anal pressure, rather than relaxation. In type II dyssynergic defecation (Fig. 4.14), there is no rise in intraabdominal pressure, while anal pressure increases during the defecation maneuver. Figure 4.15 shows a type III dyssynergic defecation, in which anal canal pressure remains unchanged during attempted defecation. All of these variants result in a negative rectoanal pressure gradient, clearly seen in the color scheme, that forms a barrier to adequate elimination.

4.2.2. Hirschsprung's Disease

Hirschsprung's disease is caused by the failure of enteric neurons to migrate all the way to the end of the bowel during embryogenesis. This condition is almost always detected in the newborn period, but some cases are not diagnosed until later in life. The characteristic feature of this disease is failure of the internal sphincter relaxation with balloon distention. Figure 4.16 is an example of such a case. While a failure of relaxation is not specific for Hirschsprung's disease, the presence of a normal inhibitory reflex practically excludes this entity.

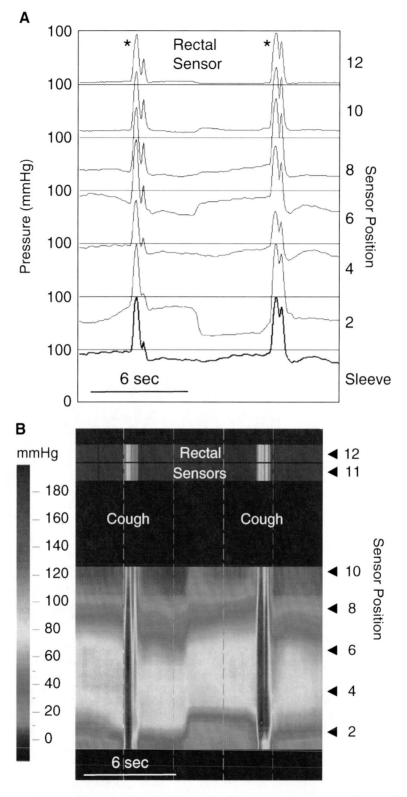

Fig. 4.9. Reflex contraction of the external anal sphincter. (A) This anorectal manometry displayed in line mode as a conventional manometry demonstrates reflex contraction of the striated muscle components of the external anal sphincter. With a cough, there is a sharp increase in intrarectal (intraabdominal) pressure (*), which initiates a sacral reflex that causes contraction of the external anal sphincter and puborectalis. This is seen as a transient rise in anal canal pressure. (B) The HRM color contour of the same data. It confirms the impression from the line-mode tracing. Loss of this reflex indicates damage to a reflex arc composed of the pudendal nerves and sacral roots.

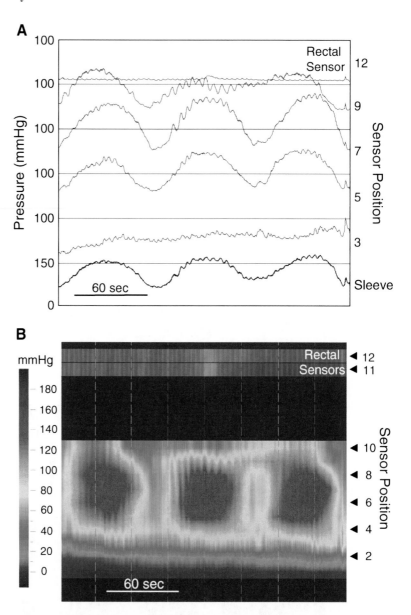

Fig. 4.10. Ultra-slow waves. (A) This anorectal manometry displayed in line mode as a conventional manometry demonstrates unusual phenomena called the ultra-slow wave. This recording was obtained at rest. Ultra-slow waves are slow oscillations in anal canal pressure that have a periodicity of over 1 minute (channels 5, 7, and 9). This pattern is occasionally seen in patients with constipation or painful anal canal pathology. (B) The HRM color contour of the same data. The ultra-slow waves are seen as slow oscillations of color.

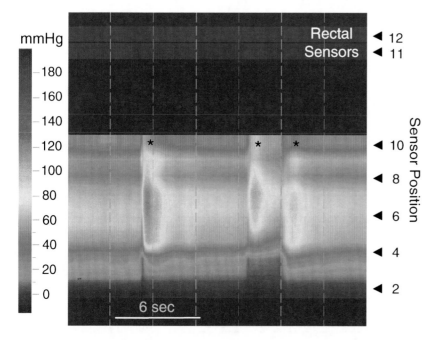

Fig. 4.11. Anoanal reflex. This HRM color contour displays the typical response when the catheter is moved in the anal canal (*). Slight sliding of the catheter in the anal canal produces a transient external sphincter contraction that is seen here as brief changes in color from yellow to red. This is a viscerocutaneous reflex initiated by stimulating the anal canal mucosa. The pudendal nerves and S_4 sacral roots mediate it. This reflex may be lost when these neural structures are damaged. Until now the anoanal reflex was felt to be a source of artifact in the recording, rather than a diagnostic tool.

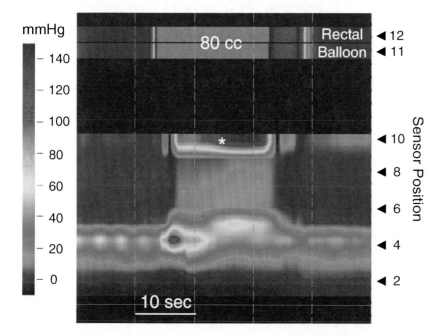

Fig. 4.12. Sensorimotor response to balloon inflation. This high-resolution anorectal manometry was performed to evaluate fecal incontinence. The anal sphincteric segment is weak and short, measuring about 2 cm in length. Balloon inflation with 80 cc of air produced urgency to have a bowel movement. It also initiated a rise in intrarectal pressure (*), indicating rectal contraction. The subject responded by volitionally contracting the external anal sphincter, essentially overpowering the RAIR.

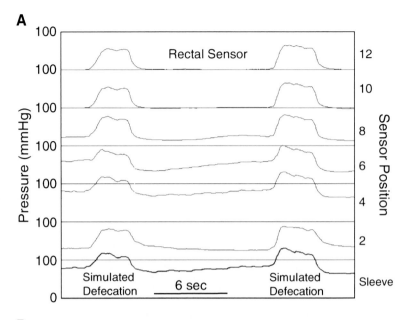

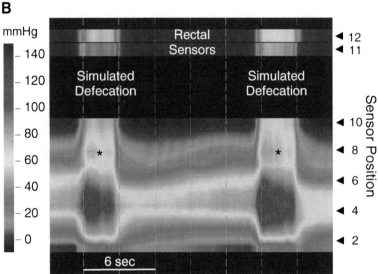

Fig. 4.13. Simulated defecation: type I dyssynergic defecation. (A) This anorectal man-ometry displayed in line mode as a conventional manometry is an abnormal response when a subject was asked to bear down as if having a bowel movement. The Valsalva maneuver produces a normal rise in intrarectal pressure during simulated defecation, but pressure in the anal canal also increases. This indicates that anal canal musculature is contracting rather than relaxing. This response has been called by several terms, including *paradoxical contraction* and *anismus*. It is now called *type I dyssynergic defecation*. (B) The HRM color contour of the same data. Contraction of the anal canal musculature during simulated defecations is seen as a change in color from yellow to red. In addition, muscular components of the pelvic floor contributing little to resting anal canal pressure appear to be recruited (*). This is not easily discerned in the line mode.

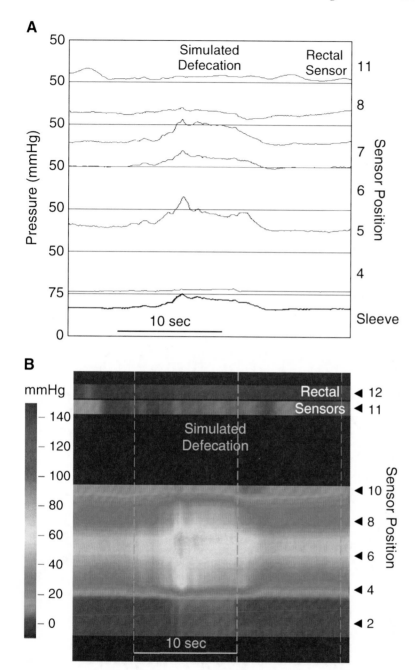

Fig. 4.14. Simulated defecation: type II dyssynergic defecation. (A) This anorectal manometry displayed in line mode as a conventional manometry is another abnormal response when a subject was asked to bear down as if having a bowel movement. There is essentially no change in intrarectal pressure, indicating that the subject did not do a Valsalva maneuver. There is contraction of the anal canal musculature. This is called type II dyssynergic defecation. (B) The HRM color contour of the same data. It confirms the impression from the line mode tracing.

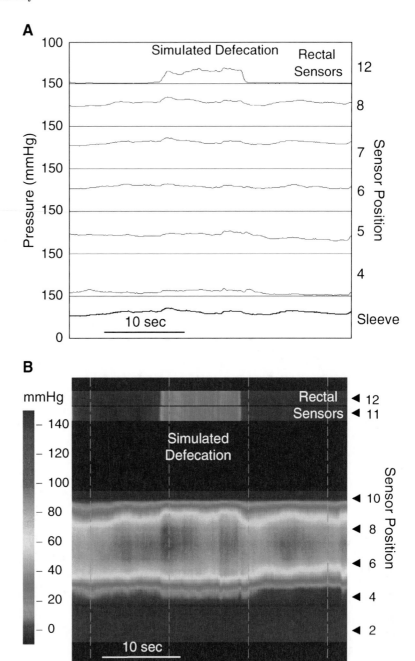

Fig. 4.15. Simulated defecation: type III dyssynergic defecation. (A) This anorectal manometry displayed in line mode as a conventional manometry is another abnormal response when a subject was asked to bear down as if having a bowel movement. There is an increase in intrarectal pressure during simulated defecation, indicating a Valsalva maneuver. There is neither contraction nor relaxation of the anal canal musculature. This is called type III dyssynergic defecation. (B) The HRM color contour of the same data. It confirms the impression from the line mode tracing.

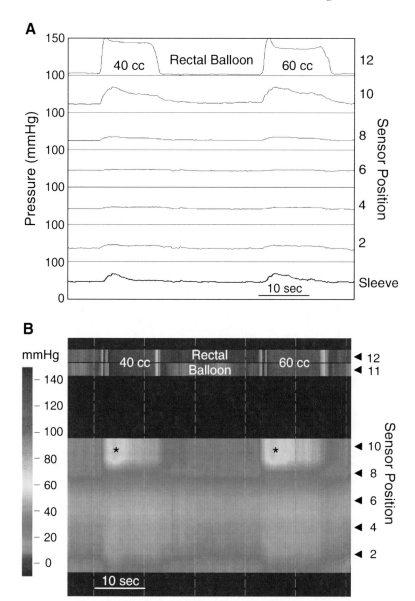

Fig. 4.16. Failure of the rectoanal inhibitory reflex: Hirschsprung's disease. (A) This anorectal manometry displayed in line mode as a conventional manometry demonstrates failure of the rectoanal inhibitory reflex in Hirschsprung's disease. Injecting air into the intrarectal balloon does not elicit the RAIR. Failure of the RAIR indicates a myenteric neuropathy of the internal anal sphincter, or megarectum. (B) The HRM color contour of the same data. It confirms failure of the RAIR. In fact, balloon inflation produces a slight rise in pressure that results from external anal sphincter contraction. The HRM contour also reveals a rise in rectal pressure (*) associated with balloon distension; in Hirschsprung's disease, rectal balloon distension can cause rectal contraction.

4.2.3. Troubleshooting

Figure 4.17 shows the typical artifact when air is trapped inside the protective sheath. The finding and the mechanism are comparable to the artifact seen with the same problem during esophageal manometry (see Fig. 2.44 in Chapter 2).

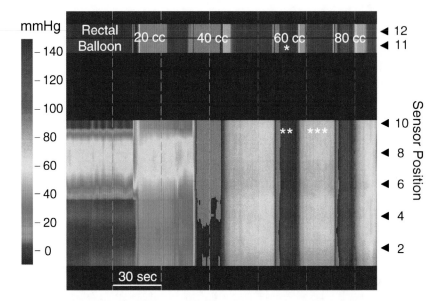

Fig. 4.17. Artifact produced by air trapping. The HRM catheter can be used with a protective sheath and balloon assembly. The balloon is tied to metal rings on either side of the rectal sensors. This HRM contour shows an artifact caused by a loose tie between the balloon and sheath. Air injected into the balloon escapes into the protective sheath. This produces a pressure increase in the sheath (**) that approximates that in the balloon (*). When the air is allowed to escape from the balloon, some remains trapped in the sheath, so that the pressure remains elevated between balloon inflations (***).

Index

A
Achalasia
  bolus entrapment, 23
  characteristics, 17
  conventional manometry, 18
  esophageal belch, 22
  esophageal motor responses, 20
  esophageal shortening and hiatus hernia, 19
  repetitive pressure waves and respiration, 21
  retrograde peristalsis, 25
  vigorous type, 24
Anastomotic stricture, 54
Anismus. *See* Dyssynergic defecation
Anoanal reflex, 80, 83
Anorectal manometry
  abnormal high-resolution
    air trapping method, 88
    dyssynergic defecation, 80, 84–86
    Hirschsprung's disease, 80, 87
  catheter, 71, 72
  normal high-resolution
    anoanal reflex, 80, 83
    balloon distention, 80, 83
    cough reflex, 80, 81
    normal anal sphincter, 71–79
    oscillating pressure waves, 80, 82
Antroduodenal manometry
  fasting state, 61–62
  fed state, 62, 64–68
  migrating motor complex (MMC), 59

B
Balloon distention, 80, 83

C
Conventional manometry systems, 4–5
Conventional *vs.* high-resolution manometry
  esophagus, 12
  stomach and small bowel, 70

Cough reflex, 80, 81
Cricopharyngeal bar, 40, 41

D
Deglutitive inhibition, 44, 46
Diffuse esophageal spasm
  definition, 25
  dignosis, 29–31
  Heller myotomy, 27
  incomplete LES relaxation, 28
  residual pressure, 26
Dysphagia lusoria, 44, 49
Dyssynergic defecation
  definition, 80
  type I, 84
  type II, 85
  type III, 86

E
Esophageal belch, 22
Esophageal manometry
  abnormal high-resolution
    achalasia, 17–25
    cricopharyngeal bar, 40, 41
    diffuse esophageal spasm, 25–31
    hiatal hernia, 32, 37
    ineffective motor dysfunction, 32, 39
    LES and GERD, 32
    nutcracker esophagus, 32, 34
    scleroderma, 32, 38
  normal high-resolution
    lower esophageal sphincter (LES), 15–16
    normal bolus pressure, 16
    peristalsis and gastric pressures, 17
    pressure inversion point (PIP), 15
    respiratory variations, 12–13
    transition zone, 13–14
  pull-through technique, 11
  troubleshooting procedure

Esophageal manometry (*Continued*)
    air entrapment, 55, 58
    failed sensor bank, 51, 55, 57
    folded catheter, 51, 57
Esophageal stricture, 51

G
Gastric bypass. *See* Anastomotic stricture
Gastric/small bowel manometry
  fasting state
    antroduodenal manometry, 61
    gastric contraction, 62
    migrating myoelectrical complex (MMC), 60
  fed state
    antegrade and retrograde, 67
    antroduodenal manometry, 65
    antropyloric peristaltic sequences, 66
    cluster activity, 62, 68
    duodenal pressure, 64
    fasting antral activity, 62
    gastric motor activity, 63
    retrograde propagation, 62
    symptoms, 69
  neuromuscular apparatus, 59
Gastroesophageal reflux disease (GERD). *See* Lower
    esophageal sphincter (LES)

H
Heller myotomy, 24
Hiatal hernia, 32, 37
High-amplitude pressure events, 8
High-resolution manometry (HRM)
  amplification, high-resolution color contour, 8
  vs. conventional manometric data, 2–6
  gastrointestinal motions, 1
  isobaric pressure contour lines, 9
  miniature pressure sensor, 2, 4
  recording, 1, 3
  water-perfused manometry catheters, 1, 2
Hirschsprung's disease, 80, 87

I
Ineffective esophageal motility, 40
Intrabolus pressure. *See* Normal bolus pressure
Intraesophageal pressure, 6

L
Laryngeal cancer, 42, 43
Lower esophageal sphincter (LES)
  gastroesophageal reflux disease
    (GERD), 15–16
  pull-through technique, 11

M
Migrating myoelectrical complex (MMC)
  antroduodenal manometry, 59
  fasting state, 60–62
  fed state, 62, 63, 65, 66, 68
MMC. *See* Migrating myoelectrical complex
Myasthenia gravis, 43

N
Normal anal sphincter
  rectoanal inhibitory and contractile reflexes, 79
  rectoanal inhibitory reflex (RAIR), 72, 78
  resting anorectal motor function, 73
  simulated defecation
    bear-down maneuver, 75–76
    catheter movement, 77
  squeeze maneuver, 74
Normal bolus pressure, 16
Nutcracker esophagus, 32, 34

O
Obstructed defecation. *See* Dyssynergic defecation
Oscillating pressure waves, 80, 82

P
Pelvic dyssynergia. *See* Dyssynergic defecation
Peristalsis
  description, 17
  primary and secondary, 44, 47
Peristaltic pressure wave, 7
Polymyositis, 42
Pressure events, 9
Pressure inversion point (PIP), 15
Pull-through technique, 2

R
Rectoanal inhibitory reflex (RAIR), 72, 78
Retrograde bolus movement, 53
Retrograde peristalsis, 56
Rumination syndrome, 44, 48

S
Scleroderma, 32, 38

T
Transient LES relaxation (TLESR), 45

U
Ultra-slow waves. *See* Oscillating pressure waves

W
Water-perfused manometry, 1–2